Congratulations

You've created your own little
miracle

THE

Belated

xx

BABY

THE

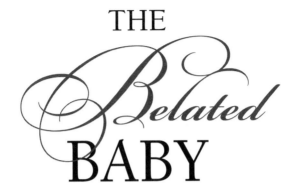

elated

BABY

A GUIDE TO PARENTING AFTER INFERTILITY

Jill S. Browning and Kelly James-Enger

Foreword by Brenda Strong

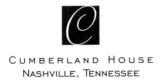

CUMBERLAND HOUSE
NASHVILLE, TENNESSEE

THE BELATED BABY
PUBLISHED BY CUMBERLAND HOUSE PUBLISHING
431 Harding Industrial Drive
Nashville, Tennessee 37211

Library of Congress Cataloging-in-Publication Data
Browning, Jill S., 1968–
  The belated baby : a guide to parenting after infertility / Jill S. Browning and Kelly James-Enger ; foreword by Brenda Strong.
      p. cm.
  Includes bibliographical references and index.
  ISBN-13: 978-1-58182-610-4 (pbk. : alk. paper)
  ISBN-10: 1-58182-610-9 (pbk. : alk. paper)
  1. Birth control. 2. Infertility—Psychological aspects. 3. Parenting. 4. Husband and wife. I. James-Enger, Kelly. II. Title.

  HQ763.5.B76 2008
  362.198'178—dc22

                                                          2008010454

Printed in the United States of America
1 2 3 4 5 6 7—14 13 12 11 10 09 08

*Dedicated to everyone who's had to
earn the privilege to become a parent,
and to our dear, belated babies.*

Contents

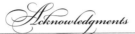

Acknowledgments

To the following women and men who endured infertility, survived, and thrived, we are grateful that you shared your stories: Amanda, Amy, Anita, Ashley, Beth, Beth, Suzanne, Brad, Carlene, Claire, Davina, Dawn, Denise, Gary, Heather, Heather, January, Jennifer, Joan, JoAnne, Julie, Karen, Kathleen, Kim, Kim, Lisa, Lisa, Lisa, LuAnn, Margaret, Marisa, Martha, Melanie, Melissa, Nancy, Patricia, Patti, Rebecca, Robyn, Stephanie, Tom, Tracy, Trent, and Wendy. Your stories of your experiences are frank and inspirational. Thank you.

We also thank the American Fertility Association and Pamela Madsen, The InterNational Council on Infertility Information Dissemination, Inc. (INCIID), and Nancy Hemenway and RESOLVE and Gina Cella for helping us to connect with so many infertility survivors.

Thank you to Brenda Strong for introducing the book by writing the foreword, and for her role as spokesperson for the American Fertility Association.

Thank you to our agent Laurie Harper, for finding our publisher, and to Cumberland House Publishing for believing *The Belated Baby* will be an asset to other parents and parents-in-waiting. Thank you both for bringing the book to life.

Thank you to Alyssa Vincent for helping in transcribing tapes and finding facts.

Jill is thankful that Kelly invaded her privacy when they first met and asked her: "Do you mind if I ask you a personal question? Did you do fertility treatments?" She also thanks her husband Tom for sticking by her side for fifteen years of marriage and during their three-year quest to meet their belated (yet premature) babies Susannah, Eric, and Will. She appreciates all of her family and friends for their support.

· · · ·

First, Kelly thanks Jill for developing the idea for the book and for doing such a fantastic job on it. She's also thankful for Erik, for a million different reasons, and Jodi and Kyle and their families, for choosing us to adopt, raise, and love Ryan; they have become part of our family, too. Thanks to Diana Gerardi, without whom this book wouldn't have been written; Finally, she especially appreciates her mom, who has been a fantastic role model both as a parent and a person, and is a wonderful "ga-ma" too.

Foreword

BY BRENDA STRONG

You don't have to be a "housewife" to have the market cornered on "desperate." In fact, if you've had any experience with infertility (and chances are if you've picked up this particular book, you have), then you know that desperation and the unfulfilled desire for a child often go hand in hand. So does financial stress, emotional upheaval, mental instability, strain on intimacy, and low self-esteem. No doubt about it, reproductive difficulties are a dramatic life crisis—one that I'm sure you'd wish the writers on Wisteria Lane *could* wipe away. Chances are you've also found yourself on the other side of those difficulties, and are now "expecting" or already in the throes of parenthood.

So the days of infertility and its uncertainty and emotional stress are over, right? Wrong. A high percentage of parents are still dealing with the financial stress of bank accounts that have been depleted by rounds of ART, emotional uncertainty and instability, and fear of the unknown future—only now they are sleep-deprived and possibly dealing with not one child but multiples, thanks to the rise of multiple births with reproductive technology and increased age. Or they selectively reduced those multiples and are dealing with the guilt of having to choose. Or they couldn't conceive with assistance, and opted to adopt. Which even *further* depletes your bank account and increases your stress, from the endless possibilities of what can go wrong during the adoption process, interviews, travel, and time "waiting" for your baby.

Starting to get the picture? Having a baby in your arms does not erase the invisible (and sometimes visible) toll infertility has had on your life. But going through infertility *does* make you a stronger and more decisive person. Every step of the way has prepared you to be a more grounded and grateful parent. Even so, dealing with the complexities of parenthood and your past can bring up emotional, social, and relationship hurdles. Understanding the unique situation you find yourself in and learning to adjust to the world of "normal" parents is just what this book helps you to do.

When I was approached to write the foreword for this book, I thought, "Finally, someone who has lived through infertility and come out the other side is telling the emotional truth of what to expect." This book could just as easily have been titled *What to Expect When You've Been Expecting*. What Kelly James-Enger and Jill S. Browning do beautifully in *The Belated Baby* is weave together real case scenarios of post-infertility patient-to-parent experiences with empathetic advice of how to handle everything from adoption to multiple births. They have combined humor, candor, and firsthand experience to gently reassure the new parents that they indeed are not alone in their journey— and yes, it's okay to feel the way you are feeling. From understanding how to communicate your baby's birth story, to nosy parents at the park, to family members who have the best intentions but are insensitive, Kelly and Jill walk you through how to deal with being treated and feeling "different" because of infertility.

Infertility sets you up for all sorts of feelings: feeling

inferior for not doing it the "natural" way; feeling superior for knowing how you so badly wanted to be a parent that you were willing to gamble your money, your relationship, and your health to be one; and now that you are, you cherish this little person or persons more than you think any other parent could. Regardless of your journey, you are here in parenthood-land, and your goal is to be the best parents you can be. Like any parent, that means dealing with your particular history and creating the future you want for your child.

We all have a different history. My husband is a Vietnam veteran, and the post-traumatic stress of surviving a war in some ways is the equivalent to surviving the unexpected mines, bombs, and shots infertility takes at your sense of security, self-confidence, and intimacy as a couple. It is an element of survival (the right to further the human race), and it is an imperative some of us feel so deeply that to live without it is unfathomable. The scars may not be as visible with infertility as they are with war, but they are there, and they do impact how you parent and partner post-ART or -adoption. Just as there should be a reintegration into society after postwar trauma, this book holds your hand as you are reintroduced to society with the "normal" parents and teaches you how to adapt and cope with the insecurities that arise because of your reproductive challenges, whatever they might be.

We are finally starting to deal with the fact that more than 7 million people are impacted by infertility. More stories are showing up in magazines and national newspapers daily. Organizations like the American Fertility Association are dedicated to helping people build families, and now even story arcs in our popular television shows and movies deal with reproductive challenges.

My character, Mary Alice Young on *Desperate House-wives,* suffered infertility and became so desperate to become a parent that she chose to take the baby of a heroin addict to save him from a junkie mother and inevitable life on the streets, only to have to fight for him years later once the young mother professed to be "clean." My character even changed her identity and moved with her husband to start a new life with their son to avoid suspicion and speculation. She was so filled with secrets that she eventually killed herself to protect them. Sound far-fetched? Not to some of you, and certainly not to me, because—unbeknownst to our show's creator, Marc Cherry—I suffered secondary infertility after the birth of my son.

We all have a journey to take. My journey led me to use yoga to deal with the stress of my own infertility and increase the chances of conceiving. During that time, I went on to help other women and couples through the *Yoga4Fertility* and *Yoga4Partners* DVDs that my husband and I produced after we taught at UCLA's Mind Body Institute.

I have learned, through my own battle with secondary infertility, that the world is viewed differently through the eyes of parents who have suffered reproductive difficulties. Because we've all fought so hard to become parents, having any "normal" feelings of frustration, exhaustion, or impatience, as parents often do, can bring on waves of self-loathing and guilt, or lingering feelings of resentment toward other parents who take their parenting for granted. Learning to let go, breathe, and embrace life as it comes are the lessons that we learned through infertility and the lessons we continue to learn as parents.

Truthfully, there is no perfect way to parent, just as there are no perfect parents and no perfect children. There is only the perfection of what life has given you, and the opportunity to grow into who you are today. That is the gift of your experience.

As you read these pages you will be comforted to know that you are not alone, and it's okay to have doubts, worries, and stress. All parents do. It's also okay to embrace the gift of LIFE your children have given you—which means there are no guarantees. I won't tell you to relax (God knows we've all heard that one). But I will encourage you to sit back and enjoy the ride. With this book by your side, you just might be able to.

Brenda Strong
Actress, *Desperate Housewives*
www.yoga4fertility.com
National Spokesperson for
the American Fertility Association,
www.theafa.org

THE

Belated

BABY

1

The Precarious Path to Parenthood:
DEALING WITH YOUR HISTORY

YOU JUST WANTED a baby.

A baby. One baby. That wasn't that too much to ask, was it?

So why did it take so long? Why was it so difficult? Why did you have to have to suffer so much just to become a parent? Why couldn't it have been as easy as it seems to be for just about everyone else?

Think back—if you can—to when you and your significant other looked at each other and made that momentous decision to procreate. Or maybe you simply finished your last pack of pills and decided to "let it happen." Whatever the case, you agreed to abandon all forms of birth control and throw caution to the wind.

It is an exhilarating feeling, those first days of "trying." You can almost taste pregnancy. Something you have dreamed about for your whole life is decided at that moment, and you are in control of your destiny. Although you feel nervous about the tremendous responsibility of caring for another human being, you are looking forward to the challenge of parenthood.

Whether you are one month into your marriage or ten

years, your heart skips a beat when you think about bringing this new person into the world. You are going to be parents, and not just "someday," but someday soon. Very soon.

Your mind fills with plans and endless questions: Who will the baby look like? Will it be a boy or a girl? What will you name it? When should you buy some cute maternity clothes? Which room should you convert into the nursery? When will you tell work? Will you keep working after the baby is born? Whether or not your questions have exact answers, the time is right to reproduce.

You were that giddy once. Remember? Can you?

Looking back now and recalling your previous state of mind (whether it was a few months or many, many years ago), you might be amused by your innocence. Maybe you now feel that your thoughts were shallow. In hindsight your passion seems pathetic. That's because despite your enthusiasm for starting a family the old-fashioned way, you've had to follow an alternate path to become a parent, one that you had never thought you'd have to experience: Infertility.

> *I had gotten married, achieved academic success, and was working in a field I was very pleased to work in. And the next step for me was to become a mom. And no matter how hard I tried, that was not going to be the outcome. It wasn't like, cool, I can really give it my best and see the results of it. It was completely beyond my control. And I really could not imagine a life without children in it. That was just where I was headed. It's what I dreamed about since I was very little. And to face that, I really felt like it was almost like a death sentence.*

> ⌒BETH, 30 (TRIED TO CONCEIVE [TTC] FOR 3 YEARS; MOM TO
> 6-YEAR-OLD DAUGHTER AND 2-YEAR-OLD TWINS
> THROUGH FERTILITY TREATMENTS)

Most people take reproducing for granted, but you now know better than to do that. What was supposed to have been the most natural process in the world—having a baby—for you has been anything but. Infertility dashed your dreams and denied you access to that elusive "normal" experience. Whether your efforts to have a child last three months or thirteen years, infertility robs you of many things besides just a baby: Your self-confidence crashes. Your marriage suffers. Your other family relationships and friendships are put to the test. Your finances—well, *what* finances? After paying for expensive fertility treatments not covered by insurance or plane tickets to far-off destinations to adopt, even the mightiest of bank accounts tend to lighten.

> *I was a mess. Mentally, you feel like your whole world stops because you can't get pregnant like anyone else. And I remember thinking, if I can't have children, what's the rest of my life going to be about? Which of course, isn't true, there are a lot of things my life could be about, but the first feelings I had, it's a horrible feeling—if you can't have children, what's your life about?*
>
> ᢒKIM, 43 (TTC FOR 4 YEARS; PARENT OF 2-YEAR-OLD SON THROUGH FERTILITY TREATMENTS AND DONOR EGG)

Over time, resentment builds. Your trust that "everything will be okay" plummets and you feel depleted emotionally, financially, and spiritually. Happiness is something that happens to other people—not you.

> *The infertility put me in such a deep depression, that I think I'm still in it a way. I don't think I've ever sunken that low.*
>
> ᢒDENISE, 45 (TTC FOR 3 YEARS; MOM TO 2-YEAR-OLD SON THROUGH DOMESTIC ADOPTION)

5

THE PRECARIOUS PATH TO PARENTHOOD

THE INFERTILITY EPIDEMIC

About 7.3 million Americans—or one in eight couples—struggle with infertility, clinically defined as the inability to conceive after twelve months of well-timed intercourse (after only six months if the woman is thirty-five or older), or the inability to carry a pregnancy to live birth. But this cold, clinical definition falls far short of the emotional devastation that infertility can create.

What begins as a medical condition called "infertility" quickly turns into a state of mind. The question is, will it be a permanent one—even after you become a parent?

☞ PERMANENTLY "TRYING TO CONCEIVE"

Few situations are sadder and more frustrating than not being able to get pregnant—or not being able to sustain a healthy pregnancy.

It's not as if you don't try your best to succeed. You have sex. Then you have more sex. Then you (both) start hating sex. You buy books, research online, talk with your doctor. You become an ovulation expert, and know instinctively the precise moment when to merge sperm with sticky cervical mucus. No old wives' tales sound too foolish to try. When you hear that taking baby aspirin, drinking cough syrup, or downing green tea ten times a day will increase your chances, you race to the drugstore to oblige.

You take your fair share of pregnancy tests—maybe so many that you buy shares in EPT as a result. You also hold more than one negative stick up to the light to try to coax the cruel result into something different. You try to be patient, but your heart is abused, strung along by the false hope that next time will be your time.

⌒Decisions, Decisions

After months or years of disappointment of not being pregnant, you and your spouse make an important decision— the first of many more to come. You are either going to start fertility treatments or start the process to adopt. Either direction requires you to make more decisions along the way, which will cause both of you your share of stress, doubt, and worry.

fertility treatment decisions

> *I kind of looked at when I was trying to conceive was like going to war. I was doing everything I could to get my body ready to be successful in my cycle: I always was in great physical shape, I was eating right, I wasn't stressed out. But the cycles always failed; who knows why? I felt like I had to do everything in my power to make sure I was doing what I needed to do.*
>
> ⌒Karen, 47 (TTC for 6 years; 13-year-old daughter and 9 year-old twin sons through fertility treatments)

Maybe you decide to bring out the big guns and solve this fertility issue once and for all. You have no qualms about heading to the fertility clinic for assisted reproductive technologies (or ART, as those in the know say). You and your spouse are examined, poked, prodded, and tested for everything from your level of leutinizing hormone to sperm motility and morphology to endometrial thickness. You undergo surgeries to diagnose the problem or increase your odds of pregnancy. You become fluent in acronyms (HCG, E2, FSH, IUI, IVF) and consumed by cycles.

Your doctor recommends an action plan for you to pur-

7

sue. As you weigh your options, you discuss the risks and consequences with your spouse. Maybe you start out with a master plan for your entire treatment experience. Or maybe you plan on just "winging it," pinning all hopes that your luck will happen the next month. Either strategy causes stress, leaving you mentally drained as well as physically spent.

Chances are that when you started your treatment, the protocol was fairly benign. Swallowing some Clomid might have been your magic bullet (and even that poses side effects). As you continue to try to remedy your infertility, though, you come face to face with your personal ethics. Just how much will you mess with nature? Maybe an intrauterine insemination will be a show stopper. Or an IUI to you is child's play—and you go straight for the in-vitro insemination, stuffing as many viable embryos into your uterus as it will hold.

While there's always a choice in how far to continue down the treatment road, you may believe that there's only an illusion of choice. You will exhaust all options before even considering that you should maybe surrender.

You're in this war until the bitter end, and will do whatever it takes to hold your beloved, belated baby.

treatment consequences

Just who *is* that person peering back at you in the mirror? Fertility drugs have the potential to impact your physical appearance, at least in the short term—and in the long term, there's the chance that they may affect your overall health. Drugs ranging from Clomid to those containing HCG can cause side effects such as:

- Weight gain—Drugs that stimulate and swell your ovaries can cause you to pack on the pounds, and iron-

LAUNDRY LIST OF QUESTIONS TO ASK YOURSELF WHEN YOU GO THROUGH TREATMENT

For people who get to be parents the "normal" way, it's about as easy as inserting "tab A" into "slot B." When you go through fertility treatment, you are faced with questions you could have never anticipated—questions you never wanted to think about, let alone answer:

- How many months of oral drugs will you try?
- How many months of injectible drugs will you try?
- Are you open to trying "hocus-pocus" alternative methods (acupuncture, herbs, and vitamins, to name a few)?
- If drugs and intrauterine inseminations (IUIs) fail, will you try in-vitro fertilization (IVF)?
- If you go with IVF, how many embryos will you transfer? Are you prepared for the possibility of multiples?
- If you hit the jackpot and get pregnant with more than one baby, will you "selectively reduce"?
- If you have recurrent pregnancy losses, will you see a specialist?
- Will you consider a surrogate?
- If you go with a surrogate, will she be someone you know or a stranger? How much will you pay? Will you keep in contact with her after having the baby?
- Are you open to using donor eggs or donor sperm (or both)? Will you be in contact with the donor?
- Will you switch doctors if you aren't successful?
- Will you seek support through counseling or peer groups?
- How much out of your own pocket are you willing to spend on treatments if your insurance is inadequate?
- When will you give up? When will your spouse give up? (Will you ever give up?)

ically make your unpregnant belly bulge. You may look four months pregnant, which invites all kinds of comments and questions—just when you're not feeling up to answering them.

- Bruises and tracks—No, you're no street junkie. Those marks on your arms are from the countless vials of blood drawn to measure your progesterone or hormone levels.

- Foul moods—When you take hormone-altering drugs, a hormone-altered state of mind can sneak up on you (and your spouse). Your sex drive has pulled onto the off ramp. Headaches and hot flashes are also common, since some meds mimic menopause.

- Pain—Painful procedures, tests, and surgeries poke and prod your ovaries and uterus, causing tenderness and soreness.

- Cancer—If you've never been pregnant and had trouble conceiving (even if you don't use fertility drugs), some studies show you have an increased risk of developing ovarian and uterine cancer, especially if your diagnosis was "unexplained infertility."

⌐DEALING WITH "CARETAKERS"

Call me gullible, but before going through infertility, I always believed that doctors cared about patients. When I had a miscarriage, the reproductive endocrinologist was callous, coldly stating that miscarriages were common and happened in one out of every five pregnancies. I interpreted this to mean that I was nobody special, and that I was wrong to feel any sadness about the loss of this potential baby. The experience with the RE left me feeling personally vulnerable and eventually led me to conclude that no doctor truly cares about my health. As a result, I'm more guarded and suspicious of my doctors and of my kids' pediatricians.

⌐JILL, 38 (TTC FOR 3 YEARS; 7-YEAR-OLD GIRL/BOY/BOY TRIPLETS THROUGH FERTILITY TREATMENTS)

Doctors come in all shapes, sizes, and bedside manners. If you are one of the lucky ones, you're able to find a compassionate health care provider to guide you through your most troubled times while trying to conceive. Even if it's just a lab technician who says to you, out of the blue, "I have a feeling that everything's going to be okay for you," you feel the kind of love that sometimes only kindness from a stranger can provide. It's those unexpected boosts that make you want to go on another day, and believe that it is worth it even to bring a child into this world—which is your whole goal!

But then there's the other kind of provider. He's the one who isn't at the ready with a word of encouragement. He refuses to send any words or even vibes of well wishes to you. (He's probably fearful that if he does utter anything, he'll be sued for failing to deliver on a promise!)

As a result, you might feel betrayed that not only did your body fail you while trying to conceive, but so too did the very people who may have graced you with some kindness to make things just a little bit easier for you. The process of infertility holds no guarantees of a positive outcome. To help calm your inner storm, you may have wanted a health professional (or two!) to hold your hand along the way, even if you're the tough type. The rejection compounds your sense of hopelessness and fragile state of mind.

When you then transition to a "regular" OB-GYN or a pediatrician, you may find that you carry over your hurt and mistrust to your new doctors. You're a bit of a jaded

11

HEDGING YOUR BABY BETS

While it's tempting to "hedge your bets" and continue with fertility treatments while starting the adoption process, there are some clear pros to reaching closure with one before starting the other. When you reach an end point in treatment and can focus on adoption 100 percent, you can do so with a clear mind and conscience, knowing that you did what you could do to find a baby behind the biological door. You can also focus your time and money toward adoption, because you'll need a lot of both! In addition, some agencies won't work with you if you're still actively pursuing pregnancy by undergoing fertility treatments.

health care receiver now, which doesn't have to be such a bad thing. You've learned to fend for your own health and not to rely on authority for everything, especially emotional support. Also, you're an expert at finding alternative ways to access health information on the Internet; for example, you can track down the facts on a child's ear infections just as well as uterine fibroids.

MOVING ON: FROM TREATMENT TO ADOPTION

I needed to know that I would be a parent, no matter what. I was ready to adopt long before my husband—like four years before he was! I think now we went through similar stages, but I moved through them much more quickly than he did. I didn't care if it was my biological child or not—I just wanted a baby. Initially, I didn't want to pursue IVF, but he really wanted to keep trying, so I agreed to do it, with the caveat that we would adopt if treatment didn't work out. Ironically once we

12

started IVFs, I couldn't wait to have "our" baby—a blend of both of us. I was surprised that I was so excited about being pregnant and having the whole pregnancy experience, and creating this little person. But focusing all my energy on IVFs for several years meant that I had to grieve the loss of my biological child and accept the fact that I wasn't ever going to be pregnant with "our" baby before I could move on to adoption.

⌒KELLY, 41 (TTC FOR 6 YEARS; 2-YEAR-OLD SON
THROUGH DOMESTIC ADOPTION)

"Why don't you just adopt?"

Even if the phrase isn't uttered out loud, it's a point of view shared by many of the reproductively unchallenged. It's bewildering to them why you would spend so much time, money, and emotional energy with ART when there are unwanted babies being conceived every day. In their (misinformed) estimation, there are millions of infants just waiting by the side of the road for a nice infertile person like you to come along and rescue them. If you adopt one of these infants-in-waiting, your fertility problem is instantly solved.

Deciding whether or not to adopt is far from a simple process. The need for a biological child is ingrained. Your obsession with having this biological baby may know no bounds. But once you make the formal decision to adopt, you give yourself permission to refocus your obsession, and move out of your sorrow and onto this next phase. Before you enter the adoption arena, you must find peace with parting with the possibility of ever having a biological child. This process can't be rushed. In addition to talking to your partner, you may want to consider talking to a therapist, minister, or trusted friend. You have to grieve and accept your losses before you can move on. (One book that's often

13

recommended for would-be parents facing this decision is *Adopting After Infertility* by Patricia Irwin Johnston; see the Appendix for more information.)

In addition to finding closure with fertility treatments, you must recognize that the adoption process itself isn't so simple. Just as fertility treatments took time, so does adopting. From the first set of paperwork to the moment when you can tuck your child into the bed in her new home, a U.S. adoption can last weeks, months, or years. If you go with an international adoption, the process can last six months to eighteen—or even longer, depending on the country, the political environment, and a variety of other impossible-to-control factors. The agency selection process, home studies, and paperwork of adoption take the place of blood tests and ultrasounds of fertility treatments.

☞ADOPTION DECISIONS

What really ate at me were the calls we got for children (gosh, at least two or three . . .) that were drug- or alcohol-exposed. Even though we told [our adoption agency] that we really weren't up for that, we still got the calls. Greg seemed to handle it better than I did . . .

14

*I just would feel so damn guilty, wondering what was
going to happen to those poor children, even though in
my heart of hearts, I knew Greg was right in standing
firm on these issues, and that it would be a tremendous
challenge and we'd have a lot of unknowns.*

⌐LuAnn, 44 (TTC for 9 years; 20-month-old daughter
through domestic adoption)

You are going to adopt. Maybe you came to this conclusion after unsuccessful fertility treatments. Or maybe you avoided treatment entirely based on physical or financial limitations, or religious or moral objections. However you arrived at the decision to adopt, you're going to face a heap of even more decisions that you may not have realized you were going to have to make.

If you're like most prospective parents, your dream is to adopt a healthy infant. You might be surprised, though, when you feel guilty that you're not opening yourself up to a wider target. There are plenty of handicapped children of all races and ages waiting to be taken in by a well-off family such as your own, after all. *Why are you being so selfish and not adopting one of these kids?* you may wonder, and you may also question whether you're a good person.

But why should you be criticized for wanting what any prospective parent wants: a healthy baby? Just because you're choosing to adopt doesn't mean that you're suddenly transformed into Mother Teresa. It's wonderful to be altruistic, and if you adopt disadvantaged and disabled children, you have put yourself onto the fast track to sainthood. You're a truly special person. But know that you're still special even if you dream of parenting a healthy baby.

You must decide from where you will adopt, but you also need to balance your wants from reality. While domestic adoption might appeal to you, the older you are the

15

harder it becomes. There aren't any set laws on how old is too old to adopt in the U.S., but couples over forty are frequently considered to be past their prime. Even so, more agencies today recognize the benefits that come with older parents, such as financial security and stable relationships. With more states recognizing "open adoptions," your child's birth mother may choose you to adopt, and age may not be a factor for her. Or it may be—you can't control what a potential birth mom will like about you and what she won't.

For many, a better fit is international adoption. There's more predictability than with the domestic adoption process (at least in theory), and the eligibility parameters, although they vary by country, can be more permissive with age and marital status. In addition, there's less (or no) risk that the birth parents will return to try to reclaim parental rights. The odds of adopting a newborn are slim due to all of the red tape you'll encounter, and the fact that international adoptions usually take at least six months to close.

Your bank account is another factor to take into consideration when you dream of adoption. Adopting isn't a financially neutral decision: costs for agency or private adoptions can range from $8,000 to $30,000 and beyond. A more economically friendly choice is adopting through the foster care system, which can be completed sometimes at no cost. If your heart can bear a possible reunification with the child's family at some point, or you're able to handle a child who's been abused or neglected, this might be your path.

⌒FROM EXCITEMENT TO EXHAUSTION

When you're out there trying and trying and trying to get pregnant you feel like there's just no plan for you. But when you do get to this other side of it, it's almost

THE BELATED BABY

LAUNDRY LIST OF QUESTIONS TO ASK YOURSELF WHEN YOU DECIDE TO ADOPT

Maybe you already answered questions you didn't want to face as you went through fertility treatment. Guess what? While biological parents don't have to consider issues like whether they'll adopt outside their race or a child who's been drug-exposed, you're now faced with dozens of questions. Some may be easy to answer; others all but impossible. But your caseworker or adoption attorney will need your answers:

- What age child are you willing to adopt?
- Will you adopt a child with health issues? How severe?
- How do you feel about the circumstances of the adoption (such as if the baby is the result of rape or incest)?
- Will you pursue a domestic adoption? If so, how realistic is it that you will be chosen by a family?
- Will you consider an open adoption (where the adoptive parents and birth parents have some degree of contact)? If so, how open? Are you willing to send letters and photos, or are you willing to have visits with your child's birth mother as he grows up?
- Will you pursue an international adoption? Which country is the best choice for your situation (age, marital status, finances)?
- Are you willing to adopt more than one child at a time— i.e., a sibling group?
- Are you willing to adopt a child from a different race or culture?
- What kind of agency should you select to help you find your child?
- How much can you afford to spend on an adoption? (Check out www.adoption.com for updated U.S. and international adoption costs.)
- How long are you willing to wait for a child?
- When do you give up?

scarier. You don't know what's going to happen and it's scary. The first five or six months of this pregnancy were scary.

I still feel like an infertile person that just so happened to get pregnant. I still feel like I'm on the other side of the fence.

—LISA, 36, (TTC FOR 2 YEARS; PREGNANT WITH FIRST CHILD THROUGH FERTILITY TREATMENTS)

Rather than being a passive participant in your quest to become a parent, you've had to be an active decision maker at every turn. You couldn't just conceive and sit back, eating pickles and ice cream for nine months. You've had to make hard choices and agonize over decisions—some of which were literally life and death in nature—when creating your family. And just when you achieved success, a miscarriage or failed adoption puts you right back to square one.

The ups and downs of infertility are not only physically exhausting but mentally grueling as well. Along your journey you may have taken a break from the monthly obligations of treatments or intensity of the adoption process, but chances are high that you couldn't take your mind off of babies then, either.

Like Pavlov's dog that salivated every time a bell rang since he'd been trained to expect a treat, how has infertility trained you to respond to future life situations? How will you be a different parent based on your experiences? For example, you might find yourself to be a more grateful person as the result of your personal setbacks, confident that time will heal all worries and wounds from the past. If you're more the pessimist, though, you might realize that your experience has made you more wary—because you know firsthand that situations don't always work out in your favor.

THE BELATED BABY

ꙮALTERED STATE OF MIND

In some ways, [infertility] has robbed me of self-confidence, but in other ways it's made me a little bit more protective of myself too. I just felt like I couldn't do anything right, because I couldn't make the baby process work for me, so up until that point, really and truly, if there was something I wanted, or a job I wanted, or something, I could figure out a way to make it happen, and in this case I couldn't do that. And every once in a while when things get busy, it's almost as if I've lost my ability to multi-task. I start thinking, oh well, there's just this feeling of failure over the whole infertility process that I keep thinking, whatever it was, I couldn't make that work, kind of permeated . . . that's my go-to when my mind starts getting out of control.

ꙮAMANDA, AGE 36 (TTC FOR 5 YEARS; 3-YEAR-OLD AND 1-YEAR-OLD DAUGHTERS THROUGH FERTILITY TREATMENTS)

At one point when we were having another dilation and curettage (D&C) with another miscarriage, we were at the hospital, and the doctor left the room, and [my husband] turned to me and said, "I don't think I can watch you do this anymore." So, I think that the hardest thing was seeing how much going through infertility stuff and the miscarriage changed me, it was hard for him to look at that. How it changed me into a much more private and sadder person. It kind of crushed some of my natural optimism. I certainly am a more private person now.

ꙮMARGARET, 47 (TTC FOR 6 YEARS; 9-YEAR-OLD SON THROUGH FERTILITY TREATMENTS)

After years of living in a perpetual state of decision-making and emotional upheaval, your outlook alters, at

19

least a bit. You're likely no longer that happy-go-lucky woman you used to be—or maybe it confirmed your somewhat cynical view of life. Living in a constant state of flux has abused your soul and changed who you are—in some respects for the better and sometimes for the worse.

Despite the fact that there's a child (or two) in your life today or soon will be, you may still find that yesterday's infertility sneaks up on you and is part of your life. Your marriage and friendships may have suffered, because there were those people who supported you—and those who didn't, making you feel at times worthless and perpetually pitied. You may feel bitter toward women who are easy conceivers and complain about their pregnancy or children; you might consider them ungrateful. You might still feel ashamed that you had to work so hard month after month, year after year, and still were unable to conceive or main-

STOP THE BLAME GAME

Are you still kicking yourself that you went to grad school and focused on your career instead of finding Mr. Right at the just-right fertile age of twenty-two? Like your fertility, time is one of those things you just can't change. Maybe you married late, or you simply weren't clearly informed that the concept of "biological clock" applied to you, too. The bottom line is that women—and men—of all ages have fertility problems, so let it go.

Rather than criticize yourself, focus on the positive aspects of delaying your family. Whether you've taken exotic vacations or have a kick-ass career, there are things you've accomplished while not gestating. Celebrate what your life was before infertility threw you a curve.

THE BELATED BABY

tain a pregnancy. Past miscarriages may still haunt you as you approach anniversaries of birthdays that never came to be.

Welcome to the "infertility survivors" club: You're someone who's learned the hard way that life doesn't always turn out the way you want or you'd planned. You learned not to trust doctors, friends, family—even at times your spouse. Or even God.

⌒BACK FROM THE BRINK

You can't be on the edge of despair and then just rebound after having a kid. Look at what a new kid brings: stress. You might sometimes believe and sense that you're especially not fit to be a parent because God didn't intend for you to be one in the first place.

You've come a long way to have a baby. Don't discount how much your infertility has impacted who you are today.

Recognize that your ordeal was a big deal. The severity of the pain you still feel will vary from others, but it will always be part of your personal history. You should remember your past and talk about it, which will validate the work you accomplished and the family you've created. You should be proud of everything you've done to be here.

Even so, recognize that the aftermath of infertility has staying power. It's a permanent part of your personality—and will forever haunt and help how you parent your child.

THE PRECARIOUS PATH TO PARENTHOOD

2

Finally Expecting:
WAITING FOR BABY

CONGRATULATIONS ARE IN order—finally! A baby is on the way. But whether you've seen that elusive positive mark on the home pregnancy test or you've just signed the papers to begin the adoption process, you find that you still have to wait for your baby . . . again.

That's okay. As an infertility veteran, you're used to waiting. In fact, you're an expert at it. First, you waited six months or more before seeing a fertility specialist, trying to conceive "naturally" and without birth control. If you went on to pursue treatment, you waited three or more cycles trying Clomid . . . then three or more cycles trying IUI . . . then three or more cycles with IVF. You've trudged down the doctor's prescribed treatment path and learned the hard way that waiting is just an inherent piece of the infertility game.

Patience is a virtue that you've had to acquire, whether you wanted to or not.

Now, no matter how your luck's been struck (whether through pregnancy or adoption), you're going to have to draw on that source of patience again. You're thrilled that your future is finally becoming a pink (or blue) reality, but you may not even realize that your fragile emotional state can impact this pre-parenting period. You're used to getting your hopes trampled upon. The anxiety and worry don't evaporate just because there's a promise of a baby. Because at this point that's only what it is: A promise. And you know better than anyone the precariousness of promises.

Managing your mistrust that good things will happen will allow you to make this time an enjoyable one for you and your partner. You're entitled to embrace and celebrate the anticipation period, just like any other parent. The question is: Will you be able to?

⌒Pregnant? (What to Really Expect . . .)

My infertility followed me throughout my pregnancy. I felt such paranoia. I never had even a drop of caffeine or liquor, and I worried constantly about disrupting the pregnancy somehow. I quit playing tennis, which was something I had done every week for exercise. I didn't have any morning sickness or fatigue, but I was very delicate with my body at all times.

⌒Claire, 42 (TTC for 3 years; 3-year-old daughter
through fertility treatments and donor egg)

24

THE BELATED BABY

An infertility veteran who's finally pregnant doesn't fuss over morning sickness. In fact, she's reassured by every pang of breast pain or wave of nausea, because it means that she's not hallucinating—it's evidence that she's really pregnant. She analyzes the biology of pregnancy, just as she analyzed the biology of conception. She knows all about it—and also has a vivid imagination for how everything can go wrong.

If you were a typical fertility patient, you took your fair share of pregnancy tests. Since you're a kind of "EPT aficionado," you might not trust this particular positive result because you know that there *is* such a thing as being "a little bit pregnant." Is that positive line dark enough? You hold it up to the light for an extreme examination. You know that the hormone HCG (human chorionic gonadotropin) that stimulated your egg production during treatments can stay in your system for as long as a couple of weeks and render a false positive pregnancy test. Nope, you won't trust this good news lying down.

Even after the doctor confirms the pregnancy, you still feel as if you're not out of the woods—you're just entering a new forest. There's more blood work. You must wait for your HCG levels to double, and then double again to confirm that you have a viable pregnancy on your hands. You might become obsessed with your numbers, just as you did during infertility, searching the internet to find HCG charts to find out if your numbers are within "normal" range. You also might be consumed by thoughts of multiples, if your levels are abnormally high. (The chance of having twins or more is increased when the mother is over age thirty-five, and then increased by as much as 35 percent when you use assisted reproductive technologies. So for many, the possibility is anything but preposterous.)

Another number about which you can worry is your progesterone level, which means more blood work. If it's lower than ten, you fret. Shouldn't your doctor be prescribing a suppository or special progesterone-in-oil injections (which hurt like hell, by the way)? If you miscarry, it will definitely be his fault, you think. You agonize every time you go to the bathroom, holding your breath as if that might stop any blood that might gush out of your body at any second and destroy your dreams. Your visual analysis of the toilet paper after you wipe is worthy of an episode of *CSI*.

That first ultrasound to see the beating heart is the hardest of all. Will there be a fetal pole? Will there be an embryonic sac? Is it a chemical pregnancy? Maybe an ectopic one? Are quintuplets lurking?

Indeed, infertility veterans aren't cavalier early in their pregnancies. It's a stressful time, and an uncertain one. They know how everything can change in an instant, and they don't take anything for granted.

transitioning doctors

> *In the beginning, I was not happy. I kind of refused to rejoice. When I got released from the IVF center and could actually go to a real doctor was one of the most incredible moments for me. I couldn't believe that I was going to go to an OB/GYN.*

> ⌒JOAN, 35 (TTC FOR 3 YEARS; PREGNANT WITH FIRST CHILD THROUGH FERTILITY TREATMENTS)

Once you make it through the all-important first trimester, you still might not feel like an ordinary pregnant person. Nevertheless, your RE (reproductive endocrinologist) will transfer you to a regular obstetrician if everything's going along as planned, usually after the eight-week mark.

If it's a high-risk pregnancy, such as with multiples, you might be directed to the maternal-fetal medicine group. There you'll be seen by a perinatologist, who specializes in high-risk pregnancies.

If you had been with your RE for a long time and felt supported by her and the staff there, it will feel strange to be "graduated to" another doctor. You might feel tentative or downright suspicious of the new doctor, afraid he won't understand your medical history and how hard you worked for this pregnancy—and how much is at stake for you. You want to be reassured he'll do everything possible to help you maintain this pregnancy.

There's also an adjustment to the fellow clientele. You may have befriended others in the RE's waiting room, since you were all in the same desperate boat. Having moved on, you start to feel guilty. Why were you "chosen" to become pregnant? Do you really deserve to be a mother, or is this just a fluke? You might feel distant from the other pregnant people in the waiting room, believing they seem blasé about being pregnant (even though they might be just as terrified as you are).

routine tests take on new meaning

> Once I got past the three-month mark, I felt pretty good; I always had that little bit of caution in the back of my head, you know, I didn't have an amnio. I kind of toyed with that, because the year I gave birth I was turning thirty-five. You know, when you're turning thirty-five they want you to have an amnio, but I declined and took my chances, because I did not want to risk losing my babies.

⌒MARISA, 37 (TTC FOR 4 YEARS; 2-YEAR-OLD BOY/GIRL
TWINS THROUGH FERTILITY TREATMENTS)

FINALLY EXPECTING

In the RE's office you were used to getting poked. But once you're finally pregnant, you might be fearful of any ultrasound wand headed your vagina's way. You might be suddenly over-protective of your uterus. Any kind of special test, like chorionic villus sampling (CVS) or amniocentesis, gives you a strong suspicion and worry that the worst will happen—that any kind of disruption will cause you to lose the pregnancy.

You know all about odds and numbers, but your doctor reminds you again. If you're an older mother (over age thirty-five), you're twice as likely to have a miscarriage as a younger woman, since you're more likely to conceive babies with chromosomal problems. The risk that you're carrying a baby with Down syndrome is higher (1 in 300) than that for younger women (1 in 1,150).

You have to weigh the risks and benefits of every test very carefully. Will you manage the pregnancy the same as if you hadn't gone through infertility? Maybe you'll want to have all of the information you can have, regardless of whether it will impact the fetus. Or conversely, will you do everything you can to protect the fetus, no matter what the outcome of any tests?

Some parents-to-be discover that their feelings about terminating a pregnancy have changed due to the experience of infertility. If they were pro-choice before infertility, they might be surprised to find themselves in the pro-life camp now. After working so hard to become pregnant, they do everything they can to protect their child—unborn or not, perfect or imperfect.

Others, though, are steadfast in their beliefs and realistic in their hopes. They know that if their child has chromosomal abnormalities, for example, they will terminate the pregnancy. Those pregnant with twins or more might agonize over whether or not to "selectively reduce." Most

28

commonly performed between nine and twelve weeks of pregnancy, the procedure involves injecting one or more fetuses with a chemical solution (potassium chloride) to stop the heartbeat. While the risks associated with a multiple pregnancy diminish, selective reduction also presents risks to the remaining fetus or fetuses. For example, the risk of miscarriage is increased.

If you find yourself in a less than ideal pregnancy situation and are being pressured to act one way or another, you deserve to find people and doctors who support your decision, whatever it might be. You must find your own path to peace. It's not fair that you're in this situation, and you might resent that you wouldn't have to go through it if it weren't for your history of infertility, but you must be true to yourself and to your partner.

☞"Pregnant"? (What to Expect When You're Adopting)

> *For me, deciding to adopt put an end to the what-ifs of fertility treatment. After two years of trying "normally," then four years of Clomid, IUIs, IVFs, and surgeries, there were no more "maybes"—my husband and I were definitely going to be parents. Years of disappointment and losses had worn me down, but pursuing adoption rekindled my initial excitement, now long-forgotten, about becoming a mommy. I finally felt pregnant—and hopeful instead of terrified. I wanted to tell friends and strangers alike. I was having a baby! I just didn't know when.*

> ☞Kelly, 41 (TTC for 6 years; 2-year-old son through domestic adoption)

The "expectancy" period you have when you adopt isn't obvious the way a pregnancy is. After all, there's no baby bulge you can point at, no ultrasound photos to show off, no swollen ankles and swaybacks that make the case for your impending parenthood. It's a secret of sorts—no one can tell you're expecting just by looking at you. It's up to you and your partner to share the news.

But in other aspects, the emotions are the same. You're excited about meeting the little person who will be your child. You may be worried that he or she will be born healthy. You're scared that something might happen to your baby, or torn between the hope that everything will go perfectly and the fear that something will go wrong. The weeks or months (or sometimes, years) of waiting seem to last forever—but any adoptive parent will tell you, it was worth it in the end.

the "what ifs"

> *I was a little unsure. There was no guarantee that it would happen, and I remember feeling anxiety about is this going to take six months, or eight months, or a year? It never felt like it was a sure thing. I was definitely excited, but then anxious, and you hear the horror stories—you know, "we gave birth and now we're going to keep the baby." That definitely played on my mind for a long time.*

> ⌒GARY, 45 (TTC FOR 13 YEARS, 7-YEAR-OLD SON THROUGH DOMESTIC ADOPTION)

If you haven't been matched with a child yet, you may wonder if the child you're meant to have will ever find you. Even if you've been matched with an expectant mom, there's the fear, unspoken or not, that your birth parents may change their minds. That's always possible. You try not to think about it, but it's always there.

If you're adopting a newborn, you may also worry

THE BELATED BABY

about the woman who's carrying your baby. Is she taking care of herself? Is she taking in enough folic acid? Is she avoiding alcohol, cigarettes, and drugs? You may feel frustrated at your lack of control—after all, you know if *you* were pregnant, you'd do everything perfectly. You'd be taking your prenatals, getting plenty of rest, avoiding secondhand (forget about firsthand—that's a no-brainer) smoke, and playing Mozart to your unborn baby. You grit your teeth and hope that your birth mom feels the same way.

And if you've been matched with an older child, you may worry about his or her history and health. What are you getting into? You worry about unforeseen medical problems, attachment disorder, and possibly even communicating with a child who doesn't understand English. Maybe you've seen a photo of your child and you fell in love at first sight—or you didn't, and you're worried about your own ability to attach to and love this little person.

You may even doubt that the adoption is going to happen. Until the final papers are signed, after all, that child isn't legally yours no matter how much you love him or her. It was just like your infertility, in a way. You've had losses, whether in the form of a miscarriage of a desperately wanted child or yet another failed cycle, after everything looked promising. You may be afraid to be too excited, to take this for granted. After all, you have been excited (perhaps naively, foolishly, deliriously excited) in the past—and look what happened.

second guesses and guilt

As you go through the adoption process, you've had to make decisions—about where you'll adopt from (domestically or from another country), and whether to use an agency or adopt on your own. You've literally narrowed your choices by going down the menu of options for who you'd like to parent: What's the age range? What race will you accept? How about health condition—does it matter? But the longer you wait, the more likely you are to start second-guessing yourself.

Should you be so picky? After all, look at all the children out there who need homes. How dare you be so demanding? You feel guilty about wanting what you want—and then guiltier still about turning down children who don't have parents to love them. Underneath it all, there may be a bubbling sense of rage that you have to be faced with these decisions—one more aspect of becoming parents that all the "normal" parents never have to face.

That sense of guilt and anger is something non-adoptive parents don't understand. Those to whom parenthood comes so easily will never face these kinds of issues, and they may not understand the heartache adoptive parents feel as they struggle with the decision to build their families.

How open you are—to race, to age of the child, to drug or alcohol exposure—is a personal decision that only you and your partner can answer. The bottom line is that whatever you decide has to feel right for you and your partner. If you want to adopt within your race, or you want a healthy baby, don't beat yourself up. That is what every biological parent wants, after all—why should you be different simply because you're going about parenthood in another way? (Just know that you still might feel guilty and anguished and heartbroken about the babies you don't adopt.)

9 months—or 9 weeks or 9 years?

We were running ads for months and we only received two phone calls during that time. One woman hung up on me the first weekend and the second phone call was a pervert in the middle of the night—I guess he was lonely and wanted to talk. We were really discouraged,

THE BELATED BABY

and thinking, "you know what—it's just not going to happen." We thought, we'll do this through December and if we receive no responses and it doesn't happen, then it doesn't happen, and we weren't meant to be parents.

CARLENE, 43 (TTC FOR 13 YEARS; 7-YEAR-OLD SON THROUGH DOMESTIC ADOPTION)

Babies take nine months to be born "normally." When you adopt, it may take years—or weeks—before you bring your child home. That means there's no set timetable when you adopt, unless you've been matched with a birth mom—and even then, she may change her mind about her adoption plan and then you're starting from scratch.

On the other hand, when you adopt you may not be chosen by a birth mom until the baby is born, giving you little notice to prepare for the little one's arrival.

Livvy was born on a Monday and we were called on a Wednesday late in the afternoon. I'd imagine if we were chosen by the birth mom ahead of time, I, personally would have a lot of mixed emotions—excitement, nervousness (mostly toward the birth mom changing her mind), sadness at the hard decision the birth mom was making. But I think it would be well worth the emotions. We got the call on Wednesday to pick her up on Friday afternoon. Thank goodness we had a bed ready, just needing to be set up in her room, and I had on hand minimal items needed to get us through a few days— diapers, shampoo, soap, bottles, PJs—the very basics.

Anyway, when we got there on Friday, they couldn't find the birth mom and wanted us to take her without a consent, which our attorney said not to do, to let her be placed in foster care until that happens, which we did

33

FINALLY EXPECTING

the next day. Then we picked her up Sunday. Those few
days were very nerve-wracking and the emotions were
running hog wild.

⌒LuAnn, 44 (TTC for 9 years; 20-month-old daughter
through domestic adoption)

When you're waiting, people around you may offer
their personal perspectives and oh-so-helpful thoughts
about the plethora of things that can go wrong. As if you
haven't thought of them already, right? The vast majority
of adoptions are simple, uncomplicated, even boring in
their ordinariness. But when most people think of adoptions, they envision a Lifetime movie steeped in
heartache where the birth mom returns to claim her child
(she is the real mother after all, at least according to the
scriptwriter) months later, leaving the adoptive parents
bereft.

Hey, nothing in life is guaranteed even with a biological child. Some women have a perfectly normal, healthy
pregnancy only to deliver a stillborn baby. But with adoption, there are more variables at play, more hoops to jump
through. And adoption is different in that you're now
entangled with the legalities of making this child yours.

Even more difficult is the wait for a child you've already
met. If you adopt internationally, many countries require
two visits—during the first, you may meet your soon-to-be-
child, but it isn't until the second that the adoption is final-
ized and you can bring him or her home with you. In the
meantime, international regulations, rules, red tape, and
snafus may mean that every day your child gets a day older
and grows a little without you.

When we adopted our son from Russia, the government
required us to make two trips. The first trip was a visit

34

THE BELATED BABY

to the orphanage, located in a truly destitute area of the country. We had to make several "gifts" (I call them bribes) to the people who helped us. When we finally met our boy, already nine months old, we spent only about thirty minutes with him. It was painful leaving him behind; since the conditions were so appalling, we worried for his safety. With each day that passed, he was becoming more entrenched in the Russian language and way of life. We had no control.

⌒Tom, 47 (TTC for 2 years; 3-year-old son and 2-year-old daughter through international adoption)

Adopting from another country, you worry about the baby's well-being in an orphanage and feel frustrated that each month that passes is another month of lost bonding time. It's another month of her learning another language and way of life. Her tabula rasa is filling up, and not with your values, morals, and beliefs.

Don't try to go it alone. No one understands the waiting process like parents who have gone through it before, or are waiting along with you. Sites like www.adoption.com connect you to will-be parents in the same boat; even an email buddy or two can help you stay sane (at least most of the time) during the interminable weeks or months of waiting.

SHARING THE NEWS (AND DECIDING WHAT IT IS)

I think it's great to share wonderful news with others. We just recently found out that I'm pregnant and told my family and my best friend. I probably won't tell other friends until we see the heartbeat. I told my family that it's fun to share happy news and even if I later have to share the unhappy news that I at least got to have them share in our excitement. Plus if something was to happen with the baby I would want them all to

35

know. I would hate to tell them that I was pregnant and lost the baby all in one sentence.

⌒Wendy, 39 (TTC for 2 years; pregnant with first child through fertility treatments)

If you've made your infertility experience public, and your support system has cheered your efforts to have a baby, sharing the news will be a breeze. The announcement seems easy enough: "We're pregnant!" or "We're adopting!" But the number of variations of infertility outcomes is infinite. Each one presents special considerations as you formulate your story for the masses.

The well-known rule of thumb is to wait until after the twelve-week mark to announce your pregnancy, since as many as 25 percent of all pregnancies end in a miscarriage before this time period. You might resent your girlfriend who recently announced her five-week-old pregnancy. You think she's foolish, even though deep down, you want to do the same thing once you're finally pregnant.

If you've had recurring miscarriages, you'll know better than anyone else the disappointment of having to retract happy announcements. Maybe you'll want to wait until you reach the eight-week or ten-week mark—any time that's later than when previous miscarriages happened. Or maybe you'll decide that since you've shared your infertility woes with others along the way, they deserve to know the good news that's happening now.

For those adopting, you'll find yourself explaining what kind of adoption you're pursuing. Are you seeking a drug-free white infant from the United States? Be prepared for naysayers to question your intentions and dash your hopes that you'll find the perfect match. Going abroad to find your baby? You'll hear various versions of the same horror story: "My cousin's uncle's brother went to [insert country]

THE BELATED BABY

and was thrown into prison for trying to adopt." People will warn you about the possible health issues adoptive kids have, or about the problems of adopting children of a different race. You felt elated to share, then dejected into feeling inferior and out of control of the situation once again—just as you did during infertility.

Those with unusual pregnancies will also face some ridicule. Being pregnant with multiples is often an obvious condition, even if you don't reveal it to strangers. You're open to speculation and jeers and jokes ("Did you have to do it three times to get pregnant with triplets?"). Your infertile past is an open record, and people will question you about it incessantly. Some are genuinely interested because they're facing similar decisions or looking for information—after all, you can't tell by looking if someone else is experiencing infertility. But some are just downright nosy and think it's their business.

Then there are career issues to consider as well. If you're adopting, should you give notice at work, just as if you would if you were pregnant? Some adoptive parents go all out, confident that their child will arrive when he or she is supposed to. Others hold off, sure that assuming a baby is coming will somehow hurt their chances.

Advances in fertility treatment may add more issues for you to consider. If you're pregnant and used a donor egg or sperm, will you reveal this fact to your family or friends—or both—or neither? Be aware that the decisions you make now set the stage for how you'll treat the truth in the future. If you keep your child on a "need-to-know" basis, how will this impact how he or she is raised? When do you plan on telling him or her?

Just as you worked as a team during infertility, you and your partner need to work together and have a plan on what your family's story will be. Role-play the different conversations and envision the kinds of reactions you'll have to your news, pleasant and otherwise. Try not to let your family's worries and apprehension become yours. You

THINK POSITIVE—REALLY!

Things may go wrong (as you know), but there is nothing you can do about that. While you can prepare for the worst, nothing will dampen the blow if your match fails. So boldly go to Babies "R" Us. Go ahead and fondle the tiny booties you wouldn't let yourself look at for years. Let yourself enjoy this time period, your expectancy. You deserve it.

That doesn't mean you should quit your job three months before your child is due, or make radical life-altering decisions right now (hey, you've already made one!). Keep in mind that your emotions are going to be running high. Even if you're filled with joy and anticipation, you may find yourself exploding with anger or sobbing hysterically for (practically) no reason at all.

have a right to celebrate and to act like any other parent-to-be.

In years past, adoption was a hush-hush subject. Today, according to the U.S. Census Bureau, there are 1.6 million adopted children under the age of eighteen, and 4 percent of all households contain adopted children. That makes it likely that someone close to you—a friend, a family member, a neighbor, or a coworker—has been touched by adoption. Still, though, you're likely to hear some pretty stupid (not to mention personal) questions when people find out you're adopting.

Decide early on how much you'll share and with whom, and recognize that some people simply don't under-

---

A QUICK COMEBACK TO A NOSY QUESTION

"Did you go through infertility?" they ask (because you announced you were adopting or are pregnant with twins or more). Or, "Can't you have your own kids?" with emphasis on "own."

"Why do you ask?" you can reply. Add a sweet smile, if you like.

Most people are good-hearted, and you never know, they might be asking because they're going through family building challenges themselves. What you choose to say next may depend on their interest and intent, but don't feel you must explain your family-building strategy to just anyone, especially if you think just being nosy. After all, no one would go up to a "normal" pregnant woman and ask what position she used to get knocked up, right? So don't be afraid to keep some details to yourself, or to choose not to answer. It's up to you.

stand adoption and may say hurtful or negative things. Educate them if you wish, or simply let their comments slide off your back. You might also hear comments like, "Oh, that's so wonderful of you!" that make you sound like a combination of Mother Theresa and Oprah—but you know better. You know that you want to be a parent—and now you're going to. And that's wonderful *for* you, not just *of* you.

⌒Explaining the Wait to Other Children

If you already have a child, you know firsthand the hardship of going through infertility treatments. For starters, there were logistical concerns. Finding childcare while you went to the reproductive endocrinologist was stressful and costly. Trying to make the medications and repeated disappointments transparent to your child may have caused depression, and you didn't want that to impact your child negatively. The older your child, the more complicated the possible repercussions. For example, maybe your daughter will feel inadequate. Isn't she enough to make you happy as a parent?

As a parent already, you may find new and different challenges depending on how you've decided to build your family. If you're pregnant, maybe your anxiety of sustaining the pregnancy is obvious to your child. If you're adopting, your anxiety over finding a match—and blending it into your current family dynamic—is also obvious to your child. (Nothing gets by a child undetected.)

You might also feel conflicted. You want your child to be involved, because it's an exciting time in your family's history. At the same time, though, you don't want him to suffer unnecessarily, or make promises that you can't keep.

It's hard to explain things to children, especially when you don't have all (or any) of the answers. First of all, man-

40

age the timing of your announcement to your child if you can. If you're pregnant, consider delaying telling them until a certain week in the pregnancy. Protect them from the hurt they'll feel if something goes wrong. If you're adopting, you might want to tell them right away so they can share in the excitement. Check out the children's section in the library for books on adoption, so they understand how their future sibling is coming to them.

The best ways to handle tough conversations are directly and honestly, and on an age-appropriate level. Children are accepting people. (Maybe that's why we're so excited to be a parent to more of them!)

⌒Preparing Your Home

I wasn't convinced that my baby was on her way until she was eight pounds and coming out of my body.

⌒Claire, 42 (TTC for 3 years; 3-year-old daughter
through fertility treatments and donor egg)

We had no idea whether or not our adoption would really happen or not. Consequently, I didn't buy anything for the nursery while we were waiting. It would have been too emotional to have a full day of returning stuff if it didn't go through.

⌒Amy, 44 (TTC for 2 years; 3-year-old son and
2-year-old daughter through international adoption)

Your head is coming around to the fact that you're going to have a baby. Now it's time for your house to prove it.

A common consequence of infertility is not preparing the nursery. If you've been too focused on maintaining the pregnancy, you might forget there will be a kid (or kids) once it's over. Those mired in the paperwork and home studies for adoption can also only imagine what life might be like with a baby in the house.

Either way, you're torn between the practical aspects of preparing (you do need to buy a crib and diapers and one-sies, after all), and the unforeseen consequences of what could happen. Is it bad luck to decorate the nursery? Are you tempting fate to stock up on bottles with newborn nipples and several kinds of formula? Many couples don't want to prepare because they don't want to go for the "un-shopping" spree if things go wrong.

You might also be wary of the idea of attending your own baby shower. Family and friends might be enthusiastic about planning a celebration, but you're busy biting your nails wondering if you'll really get to meet your baby. Just know that there's nothing wrong with staving off the party until you have your baby safely in your arms. Do what feels right and what makes you feel comfortable.

In addition to preparing the basics, you'll also need a pediatrician for this baby. Those of us who've been through infertility have been so focused on our own bodies that we might forget to line up a doctor for our babies' bodies, too. Do some research online and ask your friends for referrals. You'll need a pediatrician.

Don't let your state of denial rob you of the joyful experience of preparing your home—and heart—for your baby. Snap out of your denial! It's going to happen, so get ready, get set—and prepare for your family.

⌒The Name Game

We'd been picked by our birth parents and were awaiting the birth of our son when someone asked me if his birth parents were going to name the baby. I was surprised by the question. Why would they name our baby? That was our job—we would be his parents, after all. The funny thing was, a few days later Jodi [my son's birth mom] asked us what our choices were for boy and girl names, so that she could put the baby's name on the birth certificate. That really touched me, and it made me realize that she truly saw us as her baby's parents.

—KELLY, 41 (TTC FOR 6 YEARS, 2-YEAR-OLD SON
VIA DOMESTIC ADOPTION)

Another aspect of preparation that might befuddle an infertility veteran is the naming of their child. Maybe you were pregnant previously and had a name picked out. If you lost the pregnancy, you might also feel that this name went away along with your loss—your fantasy child is gone forever.

Was your family supportive of how you've accomplished your quest for kids? If not, maybe your plan of naming your son after your dad will fall by the wayside.

Maybe your favorite names have been taken by sisters and friends throughout the months or years of your infertility struggles, and you've felt robbed of your first choices. As each new baby was announced, you felt sad that that "Jack" wasn't yours. At the time, you had no right to protest the use of the name, since you hadn't had a child, until now.

But your baby's coming, and it's a new beginning. And he or she needs a name.

You're the one who's the parent now, and you have the right to stake your claim—and name your child.

FINALLY EXPECTING

3

Parents at Last:
HOME WITH YOUR CHILD

THE DRAMA OF infertility is behind you and the waiting is over. You're finally a parent and holding a baby—your baby—safely in your arms.

This is a stressful time for any new parent, but due to your past struggles with infertility, you may face additional struggles. If you were in complete denial that something good was going to happen to you (finally!) or worried about sustaining your pregnancy or that your adoption would fall through, maybe you couldn't bring yourself to crack open one of those "what to expect" or "how to be a fantastic parent" books. You felt like you were tempting fate by knowing too much about the subject you yearned to know about for so long: a baby.

Infertility trained you to expect disappointment, so if you were frozen with fear during the waiting-for-baby period, you may now realize that you didn't prepare yourself for the reality of parenting very well. In the words of Prissy from *Gone With the Wind,* you "don't know nothin' 'bout birthin' babies!"

If you were mired in a high-risk pregnancy and confined to bed rest, lining up a pediatrician was the last thing on your mind. If you delayed purchasing baby items, you're now scrambling to buy some of the basic necessities you've neglected to pick up—like diapers! You might feel a little (or totally!) overwhelmed and unprepared for your new and demanding family member, or members.

And then there are your expectations about the birth. If you had looked forward to experiencing a natural birth but were forced to have an emergency C-section, or had set your mind to breastfeeding and failed, you may believe that your body failed you yet again—just as it did when you were trying to get pregnant. Heap onto that a case of the post-partum blues, and you may be feeling more bewildered than ever.

When you adopt, you're not recovering from labor and delivery, but you'll have to navigate a host of other immediate and long-term issues: Will you feel isolated from other parents since you don't have a "normal" birth story to share? Will you be blindsided by unexpected health issues? Will your baby attach to you just as if she was born to you?

This is the moment you've waited for for so long—so you might be surprised that you're not enjoying it more, and wondering how you can.

ᐁFIRST IMPRESSIONS

When we got to the hospital, we stopped to see Jodi and Kyle, Ryan's birth parents, first. She was doing great, sitting up in bed eating Jello, and I was so relieved that she'd had an easy delivery and was doing OK. But I couldn't wait to meet Ryan! Janet, Kyle's mom, was holding him, and I waited until she handed him to me—even though I was thinking, "Give him to me now!" Ryan was a little banged up from delivery, and he had a big birthmark on his face that covered most of his forehead and went down his nose. When I saw it, I

thought, my baby has a birthmark. It was very clini-
cal—not an emotional response at all. It didn't matter. I
thought he was beautiful! When we look back at his
newborn pictures, my husband and I laugh about how
we thought Ryan was gorgeous—when really, he
wasn't. (Although he is now!)

↪Kelly, 41 (TTC for 6 years, 2-year-old son
via domestic adoption)

You build up the moment when you'll see your child for the first time as a grand, earth-shattering event. There will be instant recognition—knowing gazes and undeniable love oozing between you and your beautiful infant. At least, that's the way it happens on television, right?

Love at first sight is possible, but don't be caught off guard if it doesn't happen to you. If you feel trepidation when you first set eyes upon your youngster after dealing with infertility, you're not alone. Obstetricians may say, "there are no ugly babies," but let's face it—some babies aren't all that appealing straight out of the womb.

Remember, those "newborn" babies you see in the movies aren't newborns. They're three months old (at least). They don't have pointy heads or scarlet birthmarks or squinty, smushed-in faces. A newborn usually isn't a pretty sight, so don't be shocked if she doesn't live up to your expectations. She'll look more like herself and less like an alien who's having a really bad day in a few weeks.

a mix-up back at the lab . . .

I requested a mirror to watch the baby be born . . . As I
was giving birth, and as her head started to crown, I
saw the head was very dark and I'm light-skinned, as is
my husband, so I'm thinking . . . oh my gosh . . . did
things get messed up? There was that major anxiety.

47

That was a very anxiety-producing moment, but nonetheless that was my kid, she was my daughter. And there was no mistake about it. But for a couple minutes there, it was like, what the heck is this? What surprises are we going to be in for here? I was trying to recall the waiting room, and trying to remember who was there on our retrieval and transfer days [because her father was somewhere in that room . . .] Isn't that terrible? It's kind of sick to be thinking that, but it's one of those thoughts that I just couldn't avoid because it was one of those things that was beyond my control.

⌐Beth, 33 (TTC for 3 years; 6-year-old daughter and 2-year-old boy/girl twins through fertility treatments)

If you used assisted reproductive technology, you may have worried about whether the "right" sperm and egg were used. The phrase "medical error at fertility clinic" can strike fear in the heart of anyone who's ever patronized one. It's hard to forget certain headlines: A white couple gives birth to African American twins. A white woman gives birth to an African American baby and is ordered to give the baby back to its biological parents. A couple sues their clinic because the wrong sperm was used and their daughter is biracial. (Family memories in the making, eh?) These stories came to light because of obvious racial differences, so it's mind-boggling (not to mention unnerving) to think about how many undetected mistakes there could be crawling around out there.

You try to laugh off the chance of such a mix-up happening to you, but there's always the possibility that human error tampered with *your* new human in a permanent way. Those leftover fears from infertility can creep and seep in at unexpected times, and these moments following birth can be one of them. You might have worries right from the start about just who this person is, and look upon him with hesi-

48

THE BELATED BABY

tation. Even if you gave birth to your baby, you can have lingering doubts about the genetics of the child if you used reproductive technologies. Did the technician match the right egg with the right sperm? Or could one of those dreadful mix-ups happen to you?

These doubts are natural if your baby was conceived in a creative way. But as you squirm, remember that the possibility of such an error is very remote. Clinics aren't required to publish statistics on their mistakes; however, the ethics committee of the American Society for Reproductive Medicine advises that all programs have rigorous procedures to prevent errors from happening in the first place and, if they do happen, to "promote a culture of truth-telling" to patients.

If you're truly concerned, talk to the nurses and doctors at the hospital or call your clinic for reassurance or investigation. Chances are, though, that by voicing your concerns out loud with your spouse and friends, you'll feel better and see the humor in your worst-case-scenario outlook, allowing you to move on to the next worry (of which you'll have plenty as a new parent!).

divided feelings

When we found out that our baby was going to be a girl, I was so worried that she would end up looking like the donor. From her pictures, she looked absolutely gorgeous, and I admit that I was jealous. I am so pleased that my daughter looked like my husband right from birth. What a relief.

—Claire, 42 (TTC for 3 years; 3-year-old daughter
through fertility treatments and donor egg)

If your family was created via the donor egg or donor sperm route, you and your spouse probably anticipated what emotions you would have long before your baby was born. After endless talks with your spouse and working with counselors ahead of time to sort out all of your feelings about the process, you felt ready.

But there's nothing like the reality of seeing your child for the first time to know how you'll truly react. Scrutinizing your baby and wondering about him curiously is natural, which is also true for parents who conceived the conventional way. How'd the baby turn out? Does he look like you, your spouse . . . or the donor?

When the baby finally arrives, your mind may race to recall the donor profile and pictures you've seen or have. Feelings of jealousy might crop up, since you might be wistful that your baby bears no resemblance to your own baby pictures. You might be angry with yourself for feeling this way; after all, if your baby is healthy and happy, nothing else should matter, right?

If you're half of your child's genetic equation, you may also feel anxious if the child looks like the donor—but also guilty if it's obvious he has some of your features. If a genetic connection was more important to one spouse than another, you may start to feel anxious about how this will impact your marriage—or even how you parent your child.

Don't deny yourself the right to residual feelings once your baby is born. Talk it over with your spouse, and you're bound to feel better and more secure in yourself as a parent. To keep your worries buried only makes them fester.

⌒AFTER-BIRTH LETDOWN

As much as I love my friend and appreciate this wonderful amazing gift, I would venture to say that it's more difficult to use a friend than a stranger [as a surrogate]. And I'm saying that not having ever used a stranger, but, you know, in the end, your goal becomes

THE BELATED BABY

twofold, not onefold. First, of course, is to have the baby. Second is to maintain that friendship that you think is always going to be there. But then you start going through something like this, you begin to question it. And you know, there were things . . . decisions that she made, that I may not have made.

⌐STEPHANIE, 40 (TTC FOR 7 YEARS; NEWBORN SON THROUGH
FERTILITY TREATMENTS AND GESTATIONAL SURROGATE)

Now that the excitement of the big day is over, it's natural that there will be some letdown or regret. As your baby sleeps, you have time to replay the birth in your mind and agonize over what could have/should have/would have gone better had XYZ happened instead of ABC.

All expectant parents want their birth plans to be executed perfectly, but babies have other ideas on how they'll make their entrance into the world. As an infertility survivor, though, your expectations could be set that much higher and be that much more inflexible. After all, you deserve a smooth landing after the rough ride of infertility—or so you believe. Your emotional lows have been so low that you expect when your goal is finally achieved, it should take place flawlessly.

As a result of your high expectations, if the birth itself wasn't an ideal experience you may feel regret that yet one more thing didn't happen as planned. Your bodies have failed you both once before, after all, so why should now be any different?

emotional "after birth"

If you were striving to have a "natural" birth after conceiving in an "unnatural" way, you could've been setting yourself up for major disappointment. Even the best-laid holistic plans, complete with Lamaze classes and the most renowned midwife in town, can be thrown out the window when you are forced into having an emergency C-section.

When you choose assisted reproductive technologies, you're also at an increased risk for a problem pregnancy, including pre-eclampsia, gestational diabetes, hypertension, and placental problems. All of these problems can lead to the possibility of having a medically necessary Cesarean section. A mom's age ups the risk of a C-section, too. About 14 percent of first-time moms in their twenties have a C-section, while first-time moms over age thirty-five have a 40 percent chance of having one, and first-time moms over age forty have a 43 percent chance.

There can also be regret and sadness if your baby had health issues and was whisked away to the NICU instead of being placed on your chest immediately after entering the world. The older the mother, the more likely she is to deliver prematurely; for example, a woman over age forty has a 40 percent higher chance of delivering before thirty-seven weeks than a younger woman. Your head knows that medical safety and procedures win out over the personal preference to have quality time with your newborn, but your heart still wishes things could have been different.

Before you begin to feel cursed by the fertility gods yet again, though, remember that few parents feel completely at peace with how their baby's birth story went down. Pre-eclampsia, a missed epidural, or even a mean nurse can all contribute toward a less-than-ideal birth situation for anyone.

Moving forward is a mindset that you perfected during infertility. Tap that ability again and know that what's done is done, look ahead to the next stage.

birth mother and surrogate send-off

I remember hugging him and kissing [my baby] and thinking, oh, [his birth mother] is missing this. So I felt that piece of sadness, I guess, for her. But again, once I talked to some people in my life about it, I clearly realized I was not responsible for her emotional well-being at that point. It was her decision, I didn't cause her to do that. But it took quite a few weeks for me to not feel guilty.

⌒SUZANNE, 38 (TTC FOR 3 YEARS; 9-YEAR-OLD SON THROUGH
DOMESTIC ADOPTION, 5-YEAR-OLD DAUGHTER THROUGH
DOMESTIC ADOPTION, 4-YEAR-OLD "SURPRISE" SON)

If you're an adoptive parent or used a gestational surrogate, you have people to thank for delivering (even creating) your child. After your baby is born, you may have wanted to perform a grand ceremony of gratitude to the person or people who helped bring your child into the world, including the biological parents who chose you or the surrogate who served as the incubator for your baby. (With a closed adoption, though, you may not be able to meet the birth mother who carried your child.)

If the birth itself was difficult or dramatic, however, you may have been too caught up in the emotions of it all to say the perfect "thank you." When you were cooing over your new baby and rushing to phone family and friends, maybe the last person on your mind was the sweaty mess of a woman collapsed in the hospital bed. You may even feel guilty, which is normal—after all, you have a new baby, which is what you desired more than anything else. What does she have?

Now that the initial excitement of the birth is over, this may be the right time to write a letter of thanks or send a big bouquet of flowers to your birth mom or surrogate. Your words will make an enormous difference to her, and the person who carried your little one will appreciate the thought and kindness. It will help lift her spirits through her own process of recovery and the next chapter in her own life. And if you have an open adoption, where you'll have some degree of contact with your child's birth parents, it starts your relationship off on a positive note.

always a story

You may have felt nauseous hearing the fertile Myrtles drone on about their "birth story" when you were trying to get pregnant, and this probably won't change even once you become a parent. (See Chapter 6, Bitterness Isn't Beautiful.) What you may be struggling with immediately after you adopt, though, is how to concoct your own "birth story." Maybe you feel it is inadequate, or maybe you were absent from the child's actual entry into the world if you've adopted an older child.

From the get-go, you need to redefine what you think a birth story is—because everyone has one. Even if your story doesn't involve a placenta (and who really wants to hear about those icky things, anyway?), how you came to be your baby's parent is an exciting tale. Did you travel home solo on a plane from Russia with your new, screaming fifteen-month-old, encountering both genuine sympathy and scathing stares from strangers? That's more interesting (and intense) than hearing about somebody's forty hours of labor! Take a step back and look at what you've achieved through the eyes of an outsider. What stands out to you? What will people like to hear about? Take these highlights and incorporate them into your own unique birth story, which will be your family's to tell for years to come.

⌒FEELING INADEQUATE

When you go through infertility, you have time to fantasize how great being a mom is. But—and I'm being honest here—the baby stage was not a blissful, peace-ful, fabulous time. It's not nirvana—that's a crock!

⌐Rebecca, 50 (TTC for 4 years; 4-year-old boy/girl twins through fertility treatments and donor egg)

It's ironic that even though statistics tell us that as an infertility survivor, you're more affluent, more educated, and older than parents who didn't go through infertility, you also stand a better chance of feeling unsure of yourself once you finally do become a parent.

From the moment you're handed your child, you may feel confused about what you're doing and how to take care of a baby—or more than one baby. Fumbling with a car seat, diapers, and nursing may make you feel awkward and like an unworthy parent. What should feel like the most natural thing in the world—parenting—may feel anything and everything but. Your confidence level may plummet to new lows as you struggle during the early days with your child.

sleep? what's that?

Life with a newborn is one of those things in life that you never really understand until it happens to you. You may think, "Honestly—how can a person less than ten pounds really disrupt your life that much?" But days after bringing your baby home, you begin to understand how difficult and stressful taking care of a baby can be. Around-the-clock feedings, diaper blow-outs, and wailing at decibels you previously thought unachievable by a human being consume your days, and unfortunately, also your nights.

Of course, the hassles are overshadowed by your joy and amazement at finally being a parent. But then again, these hassles can be pretty hard to deal with, and they're happening right now (as opposed to that "amazement" that's taking place in the abstract).

55

SELECTIVE REDUCTION, REVISITED

There's another issue that may blindside you, too. If you made the agonizing decision to reduce a multiple pregnancy through selective reduction, the process of giving birth may make you extra aware and reflective about the loss you endured. Allow yourself to grieve and mourn what could've been, then feel peace that the baby you now have might never have been born if you'd gone down another road. This isn't an easy process, and it takes time to heal. Don't deny yourself the opportunity to feel loss and grief.

While your instinct may be to hang tough and not allow yourself to wallow or panic, you've earned every right to give yourself permission to feel tired and overwhelmed, and yes—*to complain*. True, you feel ungrateful if a complaint passes your lips, but you're not an infertility sell-out. It's natural to idealize what parenting will be like—after all, you've had years to fantasize about it. And even though you may have imagined that being a caretaker to a baby would be a piece of cake after struggling through your darkest days of infertility, it's still stressful.

Like any new parent, you should solicit *and accept* support from your family and friends. Let them do the laundry, fix dinner, or rub your feet while you snuggle with your new person. Listen to their advice on how to cope or care for a baby, just as you may have shared your thoughts to people who are going through infertility.

Just because you worked extra hard for this child doesn't mean that you're not entitled to feel overwhelmed by negative feelings. You're like anyone else who feels harried through the early hazy days of life with a baby—and just like anyone else, you deserve to experience it fully and to express yourself, for the better *and* for the worse.

energy zapped?

It's getting to be a lot more physical than it used to be; as our twins are getting older my husband's getting tired. He's talking about retiring, and I said, "And what are we going to do if you retire?" We can't travel, we can't do anything! The kids are still babies . . . our lives are very different from most people's at our age. All of our peers have children graduating college right now and are looking forward to becoming grandparents, and I feel so out of touch.

⌒REBECCA, 50 (TTC FOR 4 YEARS; 4-YEAR-OLD BOY/GIRL
TWINS THROUGH FERTILITY TREATMENTS AND DONOR EGG)

If it took you longer than you thought it would to become a parent, you're older than you thought you'd be, too. And the early days with your baby can serve as a giant wake-up call to the fact that you're just not as young as you used to be. As you shuffle down the hallway at two in the morning, your grogginess might be that much more acute when your aging lower back is screaming right along with your baby.

You may resent that infertility took some of those good younger years away from you, when you could've been more energetic as a mom. While it's justifiable to throw a personal pity party at this point, don't allow yourself. Your child needs you! You may feel less energetic now than in years past, but think of how much more wisdom you have for your child now.

Focus on doing the things that give you energy. Making time to exercise and eating healthfully will go far in returning you to the vim and vigor of your youth. In addition to paying attention to your physical needs, rejuvenate yourself spiritually, too. Whether you meditate, go for nature hikes, or sing in the church choir, try to remain true to what made you whole and happy before becoming a parent.

you and the NICU

Not all parents will experience this, but your feelings of helplessness and hopelessness can be extreme if your child must spend his first days, weeks, or even months confined to the neonatal intensive care unit (NICU). When you choose reproductive assistance, you increase your chance of having multiples—over half of the babies conceived this way are multiples. According to the National Center for Health Statistics, from 1980 to 2000 the number of twins increased 74 percent and the number of higher order multiples (triplets or more) increased fivefold.

With multiples comes the risk of complications. Premature birth (before thirty-seven weeks) with multiples is to be expected, leading to a variety of negative outcomes, such as heart defects, blindness, respiratory problems, or brain damage.

While you know that the NICU is where your baby (or babies) needs to be, it's still discouraging. It's more than a little frustrating to have a room ready and waiting back at home for your newborn and be forced to leave the hospital each day without him strapped safely in his car seat.

Instead of feeling as if the hospital has kidnapped your kid, though, try to take advantage of learning from the experts during the time you must spend there. The nurses can be a tremendous help in teaching you the basics of baby care, from bathing and diapering to the best burping techniques. If your child has special needs, the hospital will direct you to the resources and support systems available

58

after your baby is discharged. They'll also have the best connections to the equipment you might require, such as breathing machines and monitors. If you have multiples, hospital staff can establish a feeding and sleeping schedule that you can continue with as the babies come home.

You may not feel like much of a parent at first when you're home and your child isn't yet, but consider yourself a soldier who's preparing for battle. Once your baby does finally arrive, you'll draw on your NICU experience and find that what you learned from the people there will be a source of strength.

ᴥBOTTLE VS. BREAST

I think there's some guilt associated with having triplets, you know, are they getting enough attention, so I couldn't breastfeed, I didn't have enough for all three. It makes me sad that I didn't get to experience that because, the thing that was wonderful for me was that all three of mine nursed very well, I just couldn't physically keep it up. Because I would nurse, then I would pump to have something for the rest of them, you know. And then I would have to offer them a bottle because they weren't even five pounds yet, so it got exhausting.

ᴥROBYN, 33 (TTC FOR 3 YEARS; 1-YEAR-OLD TRIPLETS
THROUGH FERTILITY TREATMENTS)

The American Academy of Pediatrics advocates exclusive breastfeeding (i.e., no formula or other liquids or foods) for at least six months, so that a baby receives the kind of antibodies and nutrients that only human milk can provide. Children who receive breast milk have fewer chronic problems, such as ear infections and diabetes, have a reduced risk of disease, and show an increase (albeit very slight) in cognitive abilities compared to non-breastfed children. In addition, the quality and skin-to-skin time spent between baby and mom during feeding sessions helps facilitate the mother-infant connection. As a bonus, breastfeeding can help mom lose some of that baby weight!

Despite the good news of the benefits of breast milk, some women never try to—or simply cannot—breastfeed. Illness, mastitis, latching difficulties, and having multiple babies can deter even the most well-intentioned parents. There may be a connection between infertility and breast-feeding, too. A University of Melbourne study showed that mothers who used ART are less likely than "regular" moms to be breastfeeding their children after three months. Feelings of inferiority about their bodies may be to blame, as well as lack of support from the hospital or doctors.

Women who don't breastfeed are viewed by some as selfish, unwilling to sacrifice their bodies temporarily for the sake of their children—even though there are valid reasons why bottles line store shelves.

The guilt can be acute if you abandon breastfeeding. After all, it's the most basic way to fulfill your infant's needs. Unfortunately, your feelings of inadequacy may carry over to some of these natural activities that you wish you could achieve without trouble.

Don't beat yourself up if you have difficulties breast-feeding and switch to the bottle. Formula isn't a sign of failure. The most important thing for you to do is to respond to your baby when he's hungry, and give him the nourishment he needs—no matter where it comes from. The formula—best delivered by a confident and happy parent—will keep him growing and healthy.

60

adoption and breastfeeding

Just because you adopted doesn't mean that breastfeeding isn't an option. If you ready both your baby and your body, it can be done.

Sometimes the birth mother can "prime the pump" and breastfeed your baby in the first moments or day or two after birth. Doing so will train the infant to latch properly and provide your baby with the extra-nutritious colostrum that is present immediately after and in the first few days after birth. If that seems like a risky move in that you're worried she might change her mind about the adoption, though, don't do it. (The birth mother can also pump to provide the baby with colostrum.)

Take advantage of the lactation consultant at the hospital; she can help you breastfeed and teach you the techniques of successful latching and about the lactation aides, including feeding tubes. If practical and possible, you can pump your breasts regularly ahead of time and begin a hormone regime that will increase the amount of prolactin in your body. While it's possible to achieve a full milk supply, supplementing with formula is always an option.

But formula full-time is an option, too. Remember that no matter how you feed your baby, by breast or by bottle, the time you spend with him just snuggling, squeezing, and talking will make the most lasting impact on your relationship.

ᴄPOST-PARTUM DEPRESSION

I did feel a lot of guilt for having post-partum depression, because . . . I understand that it's a chemical thing, but I couldn't believe I was depressed! After finally getting what I wanted . . . that didn't make sense to me, and I was just having a lot of anxiety and fear and sad-

ness about, you know, can I take care of her, can I be the mom that she needs me to be?

I was a failure so many times trying to have a baby, you know, now I have one, am I going to fail again trying to raise her? I really did feel like that going through infertility, I felt so much like, and even when I was pregnant, you know, oh, here again, my body is failing, it's as if it's telling me I shouldn't be a mom.

↶DAVINA, 36 (TTC FOR 8 YEARS; 1-YEAR-OLD DAUGHTER THROUGH FERTILITY TREATMENTS)

Feeling disappointed and overwhelmed after birth and caring for a new baby can challenge any new parent. Pay special attention to your feelings and honor them, though, because you could also be developing a case of post-partum depression (PPD), a condition that affects one out of eight new mothers.

But you may be wondering how you, someone who went through so much turmoil to become a parent, aren't finally happy and at peace now. Your feelings might cause you to feel shame and extra guilt, which launches you into an even more vicious cycle of depressive thoughts.

Just because you worked so hard for this baby and your dream has finally come true doesn't mean that you're exempt from PPD. In fact, some research links ART with PPD. An Australian study of more than seven hundred new moms showed that those who received infertility treatments were *four times more likely to seek help for depression* than other moms. Being older, having multiples, and having a difficult pregnancy and delivery are all further risk factors for developing PPD.

Classic signs of depression include change in appetite, low energy, no interest in sex, and lack of sleep—which can be completely confusing information, since these are all

62

classic signs of living with a newborn! But if you're finding that, in addition to these symptoms, you have no interest in caring for your baby or have suicidal thoughts, then it's time to seek help from your doctor.

You may have experienced depression while undergoing fertility treatments, since you struggled to cope with your deflated hope month after month. If so, you may feel even more surprise and sadness that your baby doesn't instantly "cure" your blues.

However you developed depression, don't rationalize away your right to seek help for a condition that's out of your control. If you're too proud or in denial to find a solution for yourself, do it for your spouse—and do it for your new child.

ᴄ⟜ALL ABOUT THE BOND

I don't want to say it was a letdown [after the kids were born], but it did feel a little bit like—this is it? You know, because at that point, when they're so small, all you're doing is changing and feeding and changing and feeding and they just look at you—it's not really . . . you don't feel any rewards yet until they start communicating. It's horrible to say but at the same time, I really felt an overwhelming amount of love for them, so it's a very strange place to be.

All there is is just constant changing, feeding, cleaning. You want a smile or something, some kind of interaction.

ᴄ⟜MARISA, 37 (TTC FOR 4 YEARS; 2-YEAR-OLD BOY/GIRL
TWINS THROUGH FERTILITY TREATMENTS)

Creating an emotional tie with your baby is crucial to ensuring his ability to thrive. When you respond to your infant's basic needs and meet those needs, you give him a

63

sense of security and a head start in his social and cognitive development.

As a result of infertility, however, you may be struggling more than most new parents with your expectations. You've had a lot of time to glamorize the idea of bonding, and when you finally have someone to bond with, you can either go overboard or freeze.

Creating a healthy relationship with your child is a pretty straightforward process, but when issues of infertility surface, it can cause you to doubt your ability to parent well.

bonding basics

Forget the notion that unless you are handed your infant immediately after birth and let him nuzzle against you naked for several hours, you can't bond properly with your child. In an ideal world, this would've happened—but in an ideal world, you would've been able to build your family the "normal" way!

The building blocks of trust with your child are simple and they can be cultivated long after the five minutes immediately following your child's actual birth. Fortunately, even if you fumble a time or two, children are very forgiving.

Employ all of your senses to set the bonding process in motion. Touch and hold your baby frequently, and take some time to learn about the techniques and benefits of infant massage. Make funny faces and watch her reaction. Don't discount the power of your voice and how much your baby will love to hear it. Sing, even if it's out of tune; read, even if they can't follow the plot; and make silly sounds without feeling silly. Your baby will appreciate your efforts and your company. (If you have multiples, these are especially surefire ways to connect with all of them at once.)

64

The most important way to bond is just to be yourself, which will impart your own values and love to your baby. Your baby will love you for who you are more than you will ever know.

bonding and multiples

If you're parenting more than one baby, your fear of failure in the bonding department might start to multiply. The relentless routine of feedings and changing diapers and naps forces you into survival mode. How can you possibly have the chance to enjoy each baby individually? There simply isn't enough time in the day or energy in the body.

All of those attachment parenting theories feel as if they were invented for the sole purpose of making you feel guilty. When you're a parent to twins or more, you may watch that mom who's nursing her snug-in-a-sling new-born with complete envy. You may wonder if your babies will be as well adjusted as a singleton, since you can't dedicate your attention to any one baby. As a result, you feel (again) as if infertility has robbed you of the chance to have a "normal" family and build a normal relationship with your children.

In the early weeks at home with your babies, welcome all of the support that your family and friends will inevitably want to give you and the babies. Although you might resent that you need help feeding your crew, set that emotion aside and share the chance for others to enjoy some snuggles with your babies. During the times you have help, you may also want to schedule some one-on-one time away with one baby.

Just because you're denied access to some of the basic tenets of attachment parenting since you have multiples—such as co-sleeping or responding immediately to every whimper—doesn't mean that a strong, trusting bond isn't forming. Each day that you care for your babies, your voice, your attention, and your love will cement your relationship.

bonding and adoption

I had four different people telling me all of the attachment issues that I'd have with our son, since he was already twelve months old when we adopted him from Russia. With all of this drilling on attachment, I am overly concerned about responding to his every cry. I want him to learn how to get himself to sleep at night, but I rescue him every time he cries, since I don't want to make any kind of attachment issue worse.

⌐AMY, 44 (TTC FOR 2 YEARS; 3-YEAR-OLD SON AND
2-YEAR-OLD DAUGHTER THROUGH INTERNATIONAL ADOPTION)

Your primary concern as an adoptive parent is that you'll be able to form a strong relationship with your child right from the start. Without the benefit of pregnancy, you are more sensitive to the fact that you'll need to spend some quality "getting to know you" time with your new child. The early efforts you make with your child, who wasn't created of your own flesh and blood, will help him understand that you would give up your flesh and blood for him.

attaching to an infant

Many prospective adoptive parents want to adopt an infant in order to start the bonding process immediately. They want to be there from day one, or at least from the minute they meet their new baby. They realize that the earlier they get to meet their child, the bigger the impact they can have on his environment—and establish themselves as stable, loving caretakers.

While this is the ideal adoption scenario, both biological and adopted children can have attachment issues.

THE BELATED BABY

Excessive crying, restlessness, lack of eye contact or imitating, and resistance to comfort can all point to possible problems. Just because an infant is well-behaved doesn't mean she isn't in need, either. You might be lulled into thinking an overly quiet baby has no issues, but she may be detached emotionally if she never cries, never smiles, and never looks at you.

attaching to an older child

If you adopted an older child, you are probably well prepared with what to expect in terms of attachment and have a plan in place if things aren't going well. If you adopted from another country, you know that you face additional barriers with language and cultural differences. Be prepared to live your new lives together as a family on a day-by-day basis. You can't expect everything and everyone to come together harmoniously at once. Over time your child will realize that you're there to stay, which helps her attach to you—but this process can't be forced. Like most aspects of parenting, it takes time and patience.

If your child is angry, emotional, or violent, or your gut tells you something just isn't right with your child, you'll want to seek help. Diagnosing Reactive Attachment Disorder (RAD) is a complex process that can only be done by a qualified therapist. Your adoption caseworker or attorney can suggest resources that can help you; talking to parents who have faced similar issues can also be helpful.

Attachment issues at any age can send a family into a crisis. By seeking help from your pediatrician and qualified therapists, you can determine the best course of action for your child. In many cases an outside source can make an enormous difference in helping your family bonds develop and remain strong.

I'm overprotective. I tend to think the worst and the worst possible thing that can happen, and then I prepare for that.

We got a car seat for my parents' car. My husband and I both installed it, and Brad is very anal about the way he installs it, but we still wanted my parents to go to the car dealership for a free car seat check to make sure it was okay. My parents scoffed and said, "We didn't even have car seats when you were little! You came home from the hospital in wash baskets!"

So we had to force them to do the car seat check, to make sure it's installed correctly.

ᴄHEATHER, 32 (TTC FOR 3 YEARS; 1-YEAR-OLD SON
THROUGH FERTILITY TREATMENTS)

I don't want my husband's parents coming and staying over and taking [my son] away from me. I definitely don't ever have a babysitter—we don't go out, ever. You know, I want to be alone with my husband, but I won't go out for an evening. I want to be here if he wakes up, I want to know he's okay. He's just two and a half, but I'm not sick of being there yet, and I think a lot of that does have to do with that it didn't come easily. . . .

ᴄJANUARY, 36 (TTC FOR 2 YEARS; 2-YEAR-OLD SON
THROUGH FERTILITY TREATMENTS)

The most natural role of a parent is that of chief protector. From our baby's first feeble moments, we're conditioned to provide for him. That's the easy part. The hard part is letting go.

As your child grows and crawls and walks, you may find yourself coddling his every new move. Whether it's protecting him from physical pain or guarding his precious little heart so that it's never broken, you might be unwittingly changing who he is (or at least spoiling him rotten!).

Your ability to reduce the level of control over your child and let him go and grow represents more to you than to most parents, given your past history with infertility. Since your entire identity is tied up in this one person, you might lose sight of his need for independence. If this is your first (and possibly only) child, your fears that he's going to get hurt—or die a sudden death—are strong and real, and may turn you into a more obsessive kind of parent than you may have been otherwise.

Do you gasp at your child's every fall, worried about broken bones, rather than letting him climb and explore out on the playground? Do you turn down social invitations because you fear leaving your child behind with a babysitter? Of course, any parent can be overprotective with their children even if they didn't go through infertility—but could you be different because of it?

Whatever the root cause for your parenting choices, over-protection (although well-intended) can cause your marriage and family undue stress. Whether consciously trying to relax more or talking your fears over with friends, try to figure out a way to care for your child while at the same time giving them some leeway to learn how to be resilient.

⌒PARENTING WITH PRIDE

> *I really enjoyed it when he was little, I enjoyed even the yucky stuff, the no sleep, the, you know, getting thrown up on. It was just so wonderful that he was here, that it worked. And I realized what a miracle it is that anyone*

ever has a baby. So many things can go wrong. So,
yeah, I really enjoyed babyhood.

⌒MARGARET, 47 (TTC FOR 6 YEARS; 9-YEAR-OLD SON
THROUGH FERTILITY TREATMENTS)

Sure, infertility bequeathed to you some lingering doubts about your ability to be a parent, but it also bequeathed to you the most important skill in parenting: resiliency.

When you let go of your inner critic and pressure to be perfect, you can enjoy the moments with your child and the memories that you're creating together every day as a family. With your fertility treatments or adoption anxieties behind you for now (see Chapter 9, Trying Again), you can feel entitled to the same joys and frustrations that all new parents experience.

If you ever need ammo to boost your confidence about your parenting ability, think of the study that found that women who had conceived through fertility treatments were warmer and more interactive with their children than those who had conceived naturally. In any event, it doesn't matter how you became a parent. It's what you do *after* you become one that makes a difference to your child.

THE BELATED BABY

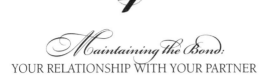

4

Maintaining the Bond:
YOUR RELATIONSHIP WITH YOUR PARTNER

[Infertility] either makes you or it breaks you. At the end we looked back and thought, if we can get through that, we can get through anything. And after having gone through all of that, it's given me a lot of confidence. . . . So the whole experience, one of the benefits of infertility, is that it gave me a lot of confidence in myself and in my marriage. It's like, okay, if we can make it through all of that, then we're doing really well. We're okay. We can do anything!

— LISA, 33, (TTC FOR 4 YEARS; MOM TO 1-YEAR-OLD
TWINS THROUGH FERTILITY TREATMENTS)

When was the first "crisis" in your marriage? For some of us, it happens at the very beginning, with a wedding. There are an infinite number of ultra-critical decisions (at least we think so at the time) to make in order to create the perfect one. How big will it be? Where will the reception be held? Will you serve beef or chicken? Oh, and (no small matter) who's going to pay for it all? The wedding itself is also the first time you must mesh with another family, so chances are high that there will be some squabbles with your future intended along the way.

71

When you look back now, though, you realize that planning your wedding ceremony and reception was hardly the emotional upheaval you once considered it to be. It's laughable to look back and remember that there were heated discussions about the seating chart or the hem length of the bridesmaids' dresses.

After going through infertility, you have a different perspective. You know now that the real crisis occurred when you couldn't start to build your family when or how you wanted. The hurt and pain that resulted from not being able to have children when you wanted to impacted you and your spouse deeply, bringing you closer together, driving you further apart—or maybe a little bit of each at different times! Even if you think you made it through infertility unharmed, once you become a parent your relationship is forever changed.

Now that you've achieved your goal and are finally parents, you may find that your history of infertility and the sorrow that it caused doesn't automatically evaporate. In fact, there's a chance that your marriage will be further strained by the addition of your children. After all, kids are needy and demanding people who can worm their way between you and your partner. (Good thing for them they're so cute!) By protecting your marriage and putting your partner first, even after the addition of a child, you'll be able to point to infertility as one of the best things that ever happened to the two of you.

↪From Patient to Parent

Whether you were mired in treatments or anxiously awaiting the final decision from a birth parent, it's tough to make the transition from the infertility "patient" mindset to that of a parent. Because you're coming off of years of being stressed out as an infertility survivor, parenting may hardly

CRISIS—DEFINED

A crisis is:

1. a stage in a sequence of events at which the trend of all future events, especially for better or for worse, is determined; turning point.
2. a condition of instability or danger, as in social, economic, political, or international affairs, leading to a decisive change.
3. a dramatic emotional or circumstantial upheaval in a person's life.

(From www.dictionary.com)

Sure sounds like infertility, doesn't it?

be the bliss you were hoping for or anticipating (see Chapter 3, Parents at Last). In fact, the first few years of parenting can be some of the roughest. Sleepless nights, a screaming kid, and stinky diapers can all push you to your very highest levels of tolerance. (You might be puzzled to think that you were patient and worked hard for so long . . . for this?)

Of course, the realities of parenting greatly impact your marriage, too. After years of being dragged to fertility clinics to masturbate into a specimen jar or having to rearrange work schedules so that he can rush to a home study interview, a husband might think, "good riddance, that's *so* over." In his mind, it's time to kick back and relax. You, on the other hand, know it's time to step up and get to the real work at hand: Parenting!

You might be more than a little confused when your partner doesn't share your same enthusiasm for the duties

73

DIVISION OF DUTIES

Women in our generation are lucky. As our own mothers (and mothers-in-law) often tell us, the fathers of the 1960s were hardly enlightened when it came to helping out around the house or with children. Today, there's nothing sexier to a woman than a man who:

- Empties the dishwasher
- Takes out the trash
- Folds (and then actually puts away!) the laundry
- Changes diapers
- Spends time with his children

When both parents pitch in with childcare and housework, everyone feels cared for and loved. What better environment for your child to grow up in can there be?

of parenting. You've encountered so much angst and drama together throughout the years that you might be bewildered and disappointed when you don't share the same level of joy for being parents. But it can happen!

Just because you're an infertility survivor doesn't mean that you're exempt from the emotions that "normal" first-time parents experience. For example, just as you had the right to complain about your pain during the waiting period, your spouse has the right to behave like a typical man after becoming a father. You had to manage your own expectations of what parenting is really like versus your fantasy, and you also need to go easy on your partner, who is struggling with the same feelings.

It might be hard to take it easy on him, since your partner might slip and make comments that range from slightly mean to fully hateful. When the going gets tough, com-

THE BELATED BABY

ments such as "maybe we weren't supposed to be parents at all" and "you're the one who wanted her" could escape from his lips. Remember: These phrases can be (and are!) uttered in any family, even those whose kids were conceived by a mere wink of the eye between mom and dad. After all that you've been through, hurtful comments carry a double sting. Try not to take them personally—or seriously, since doing so can damage your relationship.

Parenting is a frustrating business, so we're all bound to say things that are untrue or that we'll later regret. While often easier said than done, with open communication and seeking (and giving) forgiveness, you stand a good chance of keeping your relationship going strong.

While there aren't any set-in-stone stats on how many couples split up due to infertility, common sense—sprinkled with some research—suggests that it is a contributing factor when it comes to marital misery. For example, more than two-thirds of four hundred Pakistani women suffering from secondary infertility reported experiencing marital difficulties because of their inability to con-

DIVORCE AND INFERTILITY

The divorce rate in the United States is dropping, from a high of 5.3 per 1,000 marriages in 1981 to 3.6 in 2006. Everything's not as rosy as it might seem, however. Experts claim that the declining divorce rate is because more people are co-habitating instead of marrying. The divorce rate is lowest among college-educated couples, who have become flexible in their roles (and so are happier) and are more inclined to seek counseling if there's trouble brewing.

ceive. Other research shows that the more children there are in a marriage, the more stable it is.

☙Deciding Factors

> *I felt like I was sort of getting infertility forced upon me, because my husband didn't allow me to adopt. That's the hard thing about infertility . . . it's very lonely, but I think in a marriage sometimes it feels even lonelier, because the husband has these different expectations and needs than a wife does. And even if the roles are reversed where the husband really wants a kid, no one's exactly on the same page as to how much they need or want a baby. So that adds this whole extra other layer of complexity to infertility.*

☙Patricia, 43 (TTC for 8 years; 7-year-old son through fertility treatments)

Infertility is imposing. You're forced to make decisions on issues that are hard enough to answer on your own—but on top of that, you must decide each one together as a couple. Will you seek treatments? If so, which ones? How long will you pursue a biological child? Will you adopt? In all of the decisions you've faced, there's been a heavy burden on your marriage. You agreed wholeheartedly, argued endlessly, or did a little bit of each about each decision along the way. You learned more about your spouse through your ordeal, and what you now know is either for the better . . . or for the worse.

The questions you faced during infertility and the uncertainty and madness that resulted can persist into parenting. When one of you is pushy—and the other allows himself to be pushed—this can change the dynamic in your relationship, and in the way you parent. For example, did you want to adopt right away, but your partner wanted to

76

exhaust all other options first? Did you loathe the idea of using a donor egg, but were finally convinced to do it anyway? Of course, you don't love your child any less, but you might look at your partner in a different light from now on. If your vote was ignored, you might file that fact away for future use.

AHEM, CAN I TAKE BACK WHAT I SAID?

In the heat of the moment during your darkest days of infertility, you and your spouse probably both said some things that were deeply hurtful to one another. Whether the comments were true or not, it can be hard to forget and move on, sometimes even after becoming a mom and a dad.

Realize that it was infertility that was controlling both of you, and something that was out of your control. It will impact you in different ways. You couldn't fix things back then—but you can determine how it impacts your life today, and whether it will be a negative impact or a positive one.

You might find that there's still a power struggle that lingers after you're through your infertility stage. If you're the one who's been controlling and persistent in becoming a parent, your spouse might resent being the follower—and as a result, plop all parenting responsibilities right on your lap. (You asked for it, right?)

If it seems like the whole pursuit of a baby mattered a lot more to you than your spouse, you might feel serious doubt about being a co-parent with this person. Was he really meant to be a parent, if it didn't seem to matter to him if he became one or not? Did it seem as if infertility highlighted his indifference? Just keep in mind that no matter how close you are with your partner, he may not share everything with you. He may not even be aware of some deep-seated issues himself—unless he's had loads of therapy. The fact is, now you're parents—and you're parents together, no matter how you got here and what feelings you and he did or didn't have along the way.

Ideally, you've worked through all of the doubt and second-guessing before you welcome your child home. If not, you'll need to take a team approach to working out your issues—and doing it behind closed doors so that your child isn't exposed to a shouting match if one occurs. You owe it to yourselves, and to your child, to talk out any leftover feelings and really listen to one another—and figure out how to bring final peace to your family.

☞Residual Feelings of Guilt

> *I remember thinking that if I was ten years younger then we wouldn't have to go through this, he wouldn't have to go through this . . . but this is the journey we were supposed to take. You do adjust, you feel bad, and I've felt really guilty that I put him through all that, but he didn't feel that way. I remember [my husband] saying when it came time to have children, that he married me—he didn't look at me across the club where we met and say, "Hey, she's got a great set of ovaries. I want to have babies with her!" He got to know me and he knew we would build a life together.*

> ☞Kim, 43 (TTC for 4 years; 2-year-old son through fertility treatments and donor egg)

Is there one of you who was directly at "fault" for your fertility problems? Whether it was eggs that were old or sperm that was scarce, one of you may be the guilty party in your struggles to reproduce.

During infertility, you may have felt guilty for your health issues and for denying your family the chance to grow. As a result, depression may have gotten the best of you, or you tried extra hard to compensate for your lack of fertility in other areas of your life. Whether the facts were out in the open or kept mum, chances are it influenced the nature of your relationship today. One of you may still feel guilty or ashamed.

These feelings of inadequacy may continue to permeate the relationship between you and your spouse even after you become parents. In the back of your mind, for example, you may always wonder if your partner resents the way you had to build your family. Adopting from Guatemala or having quadruplets may have not been part of your Ozzie-and-Harriet dream plan in how your family would be built. You may think that if he'd only married a younger, more fertile woman, he could have avoided all the issues you've faced, and realized the family of his dreams.

Reality check: no family is perfect, even when it includes the average "2.1 children" who are born exactly two years apart. Sadly, infidelity, financial woes, and any number of other issues can tear any family apart. And while

WHO'S TO BLAME?

About one-third of infertility is attributed to the female partner, one-third to the male partner, and the rest is a combination of both—or is "unexplained." (From www.resolve.org.)

MAINTAINING THE BOND

you're not immune to these problems either, infertility probably brought the two of you closer together as a couple, so you stand a better chance of surviving as a couple—and as a family.

⌒S-E-X

> *[During infertility, sex] became a high-pressure thing. Since our son's been born, we never have sex, ever. Like, literally, in two and a half years, it's probably like less than five times. I haven't wanted to. I think part of it might have to do with the hormones and breastfeeding. I'm just not really interested, but we're just not connected in other ways, either. We were more connected during infertility treatments, you know, he'd bring the ice pack, I'd sit on the floor and he'd do the shot really quick . . . we were so connected at that time.*
>
> *You know what happened, I think? Once I was pregnant, in the beginning I didn't want to have sex because I was afraid of miscarrying and then I had the middle time when I could but he didn't really want to, and then we had a newborn.*
>
> *Eventually, the less you do it, the less connected you feel and the harder it becomes to do it.*
>
> ⌒JANUARY, 36 (TTC FOR 2 YEARS; 2-YEAR-OLD SON THROUGH FERTILITY TREATMENTS)

Those first few "makin' baby" sex sessions were amazing, weren't they? You were awash in love for your partner, and amazed at the act you were undertaking—creating a child, your child, through this beautiful act. You both may have felt important, and enlightened as to why sex even exists in the first place. "No luck yet, but we're having fun trying!" you or your spouse might have casually uttered to someone who's nosy, and asking about your plan for kids.

(Just as there's no such thing as bad pizza, there's no such thing as bad sex, you rationalize.)

But of course, the novelty of having regular "makin' baby sex" wears off. And fast. All you're really "makin'" is yourself crazy, because there is no baby! Eventually, sex for pleasure becomes a distant memory. Ovulation schedules push desire and physical urges completely out of the picture. The pressure to perform can be incredibly intense for the man, of course. It can be a challenge for either of you to get in the mood when you're so focused on the result of the deed. This can lead to hurt feelings of rejection on both sides, with both partners feeling "aren't I attractive enough?"

Even though your sex life is somewhat regular during infertility, the intimacy that should accompany it is often absent. After months or years of trying for a baby, your "regular sex" (as opposed to "baby sex") life may have become nearly nonexistent. Mood-altering drugs along with giving or getting a shot in the rear aren't the best choices for foreplay, after all. The ups and downs of treatment and massive disappointments with each one eventually starts to chip away at your emotional bond. You both start to associate sex with failure.

> [Infertility] has definitely had a long-term effect on my
> relationship with my husband, no doubt. I mean, pri-
> marily, on our sex life. To be honest with you, and he
> says it, too, when you go through five years of pretty
> much being told when you should and you shouldn't be
> having sex, it's kind of hard to get back to the way it
> used to be. It could also be that we have young kids at
> home and we're exhausted, you know? Either way, it
> sounds silly but it's almost harder to just have fun with
> sex the way we used to and just sort of you know, throw

*your inhibitions to the wind and just have a good time
and not think about anything. It's so much . . . I don't
know, it became so much more about a mental thing
then a physical thing during infertility.*

⌐MELISSA, 38 (TTC FOR 3 YEARS; 5-YEAR-OLD AND
2-YEAR-OLD SONS THROUGH FERTILITY TREATMENTS)

Now that your infertility days are behind you, the pressure to perform subsides. You can return to those passionate days of your pre-infertility stage together, right?

Welcome to passion, "parent-style."

The only thing most new parents are frisky about is catching a nap. Plus, the older your kid gets, the less opportunity you'll have for private time together. Unfortunately, sex can often turn into just one more job on the list of duties to perform. Since the activity itself is self-indulgent and has no benefit to anyone but the two (or often one!) of you, it's an easy thing to cross off the list of "have-to do's."

On top of the normal new-parent excuses for not having sex, as an infertility survivor you may still hold negative memories of doing the deed. If sex had become a rote man-on-top, legs-in-air affair, you might both be out of practice (and patience) for trying new things. As a result, not only do you feel less obligated to make time to make love, but you may want to avoid it altogether.

You also may feel less desirable to even try to have sex. If you had your child through pregnancy, you'll feel differently about your body after birth. You might find that the body-hating issues you struggled with during infertility have turned into body-image issues. If you adopted or used a surrogate, you might battle less with the physical and more with the mental aspects of desire. You might still associate love-making with failure, for example, and feel a sense of loss in the fact that your encounters will never be 100 percent fruitful, at least in the Biblical sense anyway.

If your sex life still feels artificial after having kids, strive to be intimate in different ways. Pack your mate a lunch and stick an "I love you because . . ." note in it. Pick up his dry cleaning. Rub her feet. Use manners when speaking to each other. It's the little deeds like these that count the most as quality foreplay now that you're parents.

◦ PUT YOUR MARRIAGE ON A PEDESTAL

My husband definitely feels left out, and I feel like my son and I kind of have our own special relationship and a good thing going during the week. We connect well, and then on the weekend it's sort of like . . . my husband and I are both dealing with him and him only—but not necessarily with each other, you know?

It's amazing though, when [our son is] in bed, we're able to have a totally normal conversation and feel connected. But when he's awake, it's a battle to get my husband's attention.

◦ JANUARY, 36 (TTC FOR 2 YEARS; 2-YEAR-OLD SON THROUGH FERTILITY TREATMENTS)

Although you've been through so much as a couple and held each other up when things were bleak, kids can strain even the strongest of marriages. Ironically, what you worked the hardest to achieve—a child—could be the very thing that breaks the two of you apart!

A child changes everything. Schedules shift. Careers end. Money's spent. Everything you may have held dear in the past is swept under the rug once a baby hits the scene. The trip to Rome you'd planned is replaced with a late-night trip to the grocery store for Tylenol.

Although it's a stereotypical observation, it's true that

83

HOW TO PUT YOUR SEX DRIVE ON OVERDRIVE (OR AT LEAST SHIFT OUT OF NEUTRAL)

You say you're not having sex? Join the club. Get together with any group of married women with kids (married dads, too), and you're likely to hear people bemoaning the state of their sex life—or lack of same. One recent survey of married couples found that while 1 in 4 women have sex several times a week, another 1 in 5 are only doing the deed two or three times a month. And 1 in 10 have it less than once a month. Ouch.

If that sounds familiar, don't despair. While hormonal imbalances can affect your sex drive (if you've given birth, you know how uninterested you were those weeks after delivery), lack of desire usually stems from other causes. If your libido is lagging, consider these pick-ups:

- Get more sleep. Sure, it seems impossible, especially if you have a baby. But when you're tired, you're not going to be in the mood. If sleep's not an option, make time for sex before late at night when you're ready to drop. Nap time can be nooky time on weekends, or trade your kids for the evening with a friend—then watch hers the next evening. It's worth it!

some husbands turn selfish after becoming fathers, since they miss having all of the attention lavished onto them from their wives. Women aren't excluded from some occasional negative press, either. Although she might be the primary caretaker and be sacrificing her every ounce of energy day in and day out to her child, a mother's not doing her marriage any favors by focusing so much on her child. There's nothing less attractive to a man (or anyone) than a perpetual martyr.

84

- Hit the gym. Regular exercise, including yoga, helps you manage stress, gives you more energy, and improves the look of your body—plus how sexy and confident you feel.
- Eat more fruits and veggies. A nutritious diet gives you the energy and stamina you need between the sheets. But don't slash your caloric intake too drastically to lose weight—women on diets tend to feel cranky, tired, and uninterested in anything but food!
- Talk to your doctor. If your lack of desire persists, there may be a medical reason such as depression or hypothyroidism at play. And some drugs, including antidepressants, can also affect sexual desire.
- Connect with your partner. Often lack of desire stems from resentment or unresolved issues—and skipping or avoiding sex only makes matters worse. There's nothing wrong with an occasional "by rote" romp to keep that connection strong. Sex and the intimacy afterwards is one of the glues that holds your relationship together, so don't always feel that you have to be in the mood. Sometimes once you start, you *get* in the mood!

As an infertility survivor, it might be even harder for you to allow your child to find some independence out in the real world. You might have an even stronger sense of wanting to shelter your child since you worked so hard to have him. If you adopt, you might feel an extra layer of obligation to take extra care of the child, since you are the steward of the child on behalf of so many other people who care about him.

When you put your child above all others, though, you

85

TIME FOR COUNSELING?

Do you and your spouse fight constructively, or does it seem like you're both about to self-destruct? Whether you're repeating arguments without a resolution in sight, shout frequently and in front of the kids, or feel trapped by the whole situation, it might be time to seek a therapist for help. There's no need to feel ashamed to ask for help, which might be covered by your insurance.

run the risk of short-changing your child in the end. If his needs are always put above those of yours and your spouse, he soon learns that he's the one running this family's show. Do you really want that kid living with you in ten years?

Do your marriage a favor, and protect it from being permanently damaged by your children. Create a united front to your child, and boundaries within your own relationship that pledge to honor your own bond together.

⌒ Time Is (Finally!) on Your Side

A lot of times people get married, and within a couple of years they're having kids, you know. I think for better or worse my husband and I had a lot of years alone together. Sometimes we miss our alone time, don't get me wrong, but it's never like, it's not like we feel like kids came too soon or that we didn't have enough time to ourselves to do things.

~ JoAnne, 37 (TTC for 4 years; 3-year-old daughter and 5-month-old son through fertility treatments)

As an infertility survivor, you may lament the fact that you had a late start in the baby-building game. Blame it on your career, a laid-back gynecologist ("you're too young to worry about starting a family," she said), or ignorance that as you age it would be harder to conceive. The bottom line is that you probably were blindsided that infertility could possibly happen to you.

As you tried to conceive, time passed. Then more time passed. How did you fill that time, waiting for your tardy baby? Spending time with your spouse, no doubt! The two of you dedicated endless hours talking and agonizing over what your next baby-obtaining moves would be. You drove an hour each way to sit in a waiting room together, holding hands, anxious for the next piece of news or diagnosis. You researched adoption topics online together. To lighten your moods and cheer one another up, you shopped or rode bikes or went out to lunch . . . and tried not to cry when the host seated a couple with a newborn right next to your table.

In addition to the quality time (with a helping of emotional turmoil) you spent together pre-kid, you were physically exposed to one another during infertility, too. Forced sex, ultrasound after ultrasound, HCG shots, laparoscopy.

NOT OPTIONAL: MAKING "DATE NIGHTS" A PRIORITY

While you were waiting to be parents, what did you do together to blow off steam? Whether it was going for a walk, to the movies, or skydiving, make time for these activities after you become parents, too. It might be hard to break away from your child since you waited so long to have him, but it's crucial to nurture your marriage just as much as you do your child.

MAINTAINING THE BOND

BABYSITTER, 911!

Are you using the excuse that you can't find a sitter as the reason you can't find time for yourself? Finding childcare isn't as difficult as you think, if you're willing to be creative. Search out the teens in your neighborhood, or post a "help wanted" flier up on the community college bulletin board. Sure, you might not leave your eight-month-old with a twelve-year-old. But you could hire her as a "mother's helper." While you fold laundry, fix dinner, or hide upstairs with a novel, she can play with your baby. Don't feel guilty about it either: Your child will benefit from hanging out with someone other than you.

Also consider letting your spouse take care of things solo for a full day, if you're the one who's normally in charge. Let him run the show for once, and without a running commentary from you on how he's doing everything wrong. (Strive to self-edit, which, admittedly, is much, much easier said than done.)

You both might have felt like senior citizens, you visited the doctor so often! The entire experience caused you both to be exposed to one another fully, in a real and raw way.

While you're done with the doctor, remember that spending time in and out of bed together is an excellent prescription for happiness for any couple—whether they're going through infertility or not. Try to remember how you nurtured each other as individuals throughout infertility and consider it as an investment—because these same moves work for taking care of yourselves as parents, too!

Celebrate the time you had together pre-kids, and consider it a lesson in how to be a united front for your new family.

◦Newfound Respect

Obviously, I was always very attracted to my wife and we were very similar and had a lot of the same values. But going through infertility, I was amazed by her determination and drive to become a mom. It was seeing a whole other side of her that I really responded to.

◦Trent, 35 (TTC for 2 years; infant boy/girl twins through fertility treatments)

The two of you have seen things about each other, physically and emotionally, that you never had witnessed before infertility, and might not have even after infertility—if you're lucky. You encountered the full spectrum of emotions together, from the highs of receiving a positive pregnancy test to the lows of a devastating miscarriage.

How did you act when faced with horrible news? Were you an optimist, always ready to bounce back? Or did you sink to new, never-before-recorded lows, unable to deal? What about your spouse?

Having gone through infertility, your spouse couldn't help but view you in a different light. Your husband's heart broke when he saw you in pain, either huddled in a corner crying your eyes out or slumped in a hospital bed awaiting your third D&C. You pitied his defeated looks and frustrated shrugs every time a negative test popped up. You both admire the effort and significance of what each of you has done to build your family—from the painful infertility tests to the exuberant action of signing on the adoption agency contract's bottom line.

Chances are that you took turns acting crazed, angry, and calm—ideally at different times—and that's what made

89

the experience tolerable. You balanced each other out and took turns being uplifting; one stayed strong while the other one felt weak. You are like war buddies who've seen combat and survived it together. As a result, the bond you share is probably stronger than ever, and ready to face the challenge of parenting . . . a new kind of war. (Difficult, but far, far easier than infertility!)

⌒STRONG FATHERS

> *I mean, it's not a huge difference, but [fathers who've been through infertility] are just a little bit more involved. I don't think they have as much of a tendency to take parenting for granted. And it could just be it's a level of maturity too, and maybe the people who had kids come earlier, I mean, maybe they were younger . . . and men kind of take longer to mature, so maybe they had kids in their twenties when they weren't quite ready. But maybe when a guy is in his thirties he's a little more ready to stop hanging out with the guys and be at home with his kids.*

> ⌒JOANNE, 37 (TTC FOR 4 YEARS; 3-YEAR-OLD DAUGHTER AND
> 5-MONTH-OLD SON THROUGH FERTILITY TREATMENTS)

While the stereotype is that new fathers are sulking, pouting people who feel ignored and overshadowed by the baby, just the opposite may be true for those of us who've made it through infertility. These are the men who realize more acutely the miracle of children, and don't take it for granted once they finally become fathers.

Think about it: Dads who reproduce the regular way have it relatively easy. They sow their oats, then sit back and let their wives takes care of the details of gestating. Those who go through infertility, on the other hand, see it all. They see their sperm. They see the ultrasounds beaming

90

back uterine linings and ripe follicles. They become as well-versed as any woman with the terminology of infertility, the measurements and science of it all. They're active participants in the creation of their families, whether it happens at the clinic or at the adoption agency. They're involved and invested in their kids—even before they meet them.

All sunshine makes a desert.

⌐ARAB PROVERB

From changing diapers to taking a toddler out to breakfast solo, it's impossible (and possibly unfair to all other superb dads out there, of which there are many!) to directly relate a dad's every action back to his infertility experience. At the same time, it's also impossible to believe that infertility didn't shape his current behavior and attitude at all. Sure, you can be a fantastic father without ever going through a single day of infertility angst. But as an infertility survivor, there must be something positive somewhere in the experience . . . and having a smidge more of "fantasticness" might well be one of them!

⌐INFERTILITY: THE ULTIMATE MARRIAGE CHARACTER-BUILDER

> We don't have to wait until ten years from now into our marriage to know if we can handle something. Say that we have a child that's disabled in some way, or let's say we have a child that gets really sick and needs like a transplant or something crazy like that . . . I'm just thinking anything really bad, those terrible things that can happen where it can take a stress on your marriage.
>
> We're 100 percent sure that we're going to be able to pull through just about anything at this point. And it's just good to know that. . . . So, despite all the pain and

91

frustration, and all that stuff, I think that something good has come out of it, and that's the peace of mind knowing that what we have is something really good, really special.

⌐Lisa, 36, (TTC for 2 years; pregnant with first child through fertility treatments)

Imagine for a moment that you and your spouse never had to deal with infertility. Instead of being thwarted at every baby-making turn, you were able to get pregnant the first month you tried and then sail through pregnancy and give birth like a normal couple. Of course, your babies were spaced perfectly two years apart—just as you had planned. Like clockwork, everything fell into place.

In this fantasy scenario, is the relationship between the two of you different than it is today? Is it better? Worse? How did infertility change you? Would you trade your marriage for that one?

No matter what your answers are, there's no doubt that you've grown personally through your turmoil. Your priorities, values, and respect for one another have developed, and a connection between the two of you is stronger. Just as a dispute over the flavor of your wedding cake no longer constitutes a crisis, neither does who's changed more diapers to date—you or your spouse. You're more of an adult.

You recognize infertility as a blessing in your life. Not only because it has given you the child you're caring for today, but because it's brought your marriage to a higher level of understanding and love. You've survived it together!

THE BELATED BABY

5

Family Ties:
HOW YOUR RELATIONSHIPS CHANGE

[My family] was very supportive. By all means they were very understanding, but at the same time, they weren't. They would definitely pull me aside sometimes and be like, "Listen, you can't think about [infertility] constantly." They would say, "We're trying to understand and we're sorry . . . but at the same time, we want to see you thinking and talking about something else and enjoying other things in life, rather than where you are in your cycle and when your next appointment is." They were sick of hearing about our infertility.

                          ⌒MELISSA, 38 (TTC FOR 3 YEARS; 5-YEAR-OLD AND
                          2-YEAR-OLD SONS THROUGH FERTILITY TREATMENTS)

Going through infertility wasn't just a crisis for you and your partner, you know. It also stressed out many of the people who love you. As you anguished, so did family and friends.

Now that you're a parent (or soon will be), it might be easier for you to understand how your loved ones felt, watching you go through all of the hell, hurt, and pain of trying to grow your family. You already know, or have some inkling, of the lengths you'd go to in order to protect your own child from experiencing any deep heartache. Well, your parents feel the same way about you. Maybe they knew just how to comfort you, or at least tried to. Or maybe they simply withdrew, unsure of what to say or how to help.

Whether your family is delightful or dysfunctional—or a bit of both—they're part of who you are and your personal history. They may also be part of the reason why you wanted to become a parent so much in the first place. Whether they taught you about the true value and meaning of family firsthand or inspired you to improve on what they failed to create, you learned many lessons about family from your family.

And no matter how complicated your relationship with your family is, you probably do care about what they think. Before infertility took hold, you may have conjured up all sorts of fun ways to tell them that you were pregnant. Gathered around the Thanksgiving table with aunts, uncles, cousins, and grandma, you were going to proclaim that you were due in June—surprise! "Oooh!" They would clap. Or the news would be given as a playful prank, maybe with a diaper stuck in your mom's purse. "What's this?" she'd ask. You'd laugh and spring the news. Surprise—you're due in August! "Aaah!" She'd give you a big hug and touch your tummy lovingly. She'd be so proud.

But things didn't go down that way, of course. As time passed and infertility took hold, your fantasies of how you would tell your family faded—one of the first casualties of infertility. If you did finally manage to get pregnant, you probably delivered the news quietly . . . cautiously. Conditioned to expect bad outcomes, you knew not to get your hopes up too high. You were sensitive, and you wanted to manage your family's expectations, too.

94

Were family and friends supportive of your efforts to become parents? If so, you'll continue to draw from their experience and love, which will help you be the best

In prosperity our friends know us; in adversity we know our friends.

—JOHN CHURTON COLLINS
(LITERARY CRITIC, 1848–1908)

parent possible. If they weren't supportive or if you felt criticized after key decisions you were forced to make, you may have unresolved feelings—of anger, envy, even spite— that may affect your relationship with those closest to you.

Your family's attitude toward you and your child or children cannot be discounted, but sometimes it can't be changed either. If you and your family members can't stay connected or reconnect once you're a parent, chances are it might be time to cut ties . . . or at least slash your expectations of those you love.

DURING THE IF INFERNO

[My mom was supportive of us trying to have a baby], but by the time we got to the IVF, she was very much like, 'I don't want you to do this, this is too dangerous. I would never do this.' Still to this day, she talks to the boys and is like, 'Your mommy went through so much to get you, and I would never have done that to get you, but your mommy went through so much to get you.'

—HEATHER, 33 (TTC FOR 5 YEARS; 1-YEAR-OLD TWIN BOYS)

You know your family wants the best for you, and your confidence that they wanted things to work out during infertility may have never wavered. Even so, some families have a funny way of showing love and support—because their darn personalities and opinions tend to get in the way.

In the beginning, before they knew your full story, family members may have unwittingly asked cruel questions or made insensitive comments. When are you going to make them a grandma, grandpa, aunt, or uncle? Why are you working so hard on your career instead of starting a family? What's taking so long—do you even know how babies are made?

If you "came clean" about the infertility, the badgering may have continued. What about wearing boxers? Did you see the promising news about acupuncture? Are you seeing the best doctor? Are you at least *trying* to relax? (Then you'll get pregnant for sure.) The questioning may have turned into smothering, and you had to report news on an hourly basis—even if it was just "there is no news." Or, they may have avoided the issue altogether, choosing to talk about sports, the lawn, or the cold front headed your way instead.

As your efforts progressed, the caring from your family may not have always come in the form that you'd hoped it would. After you just found out about a failed cycle, your eternal optimist dad started delivering a pick-me-up speech . . . when all you craved was a hug. You were encouraged by a promising lead on a birth mother, which prompted your sister to recount a lengthy (and quite inaccurate) version of the "baby Richard" case. Not quite over the Cold War herself, your mother sat, silently stoic, while you told her you and your partner were heading to Russia.

No one's perfect, you realize. Boundaries were overstepped. Pitiful looks given. Whether your family was optimistic or pessimistic, loose-lipped or quiet as church mice, you forgave them for their missteps. Or maybe you haven't.

judgment days

What makes forgiving and forgetting especially difficult, though, is if your family was opposed to your efforts from the start. If you and your same-sex partner spent countless dollars on IVF cycles, maybe your family didn't understand

96

your fundamental desire to become parents. (Well, maybe they also don't understand your desire for one another—but that's another story!) If you knew you could tackle single motherhood, your conservative brother might have disagreed and disavowed your pursuit. Was Uncle Bob opposed to ART based on religious reasons? Then you weren't entitled to feel frustrated by another negative pregnancy test.

Whether you skipped treatments altogether or reached the point of saying "enough!" to the never-ending rounds of

---

HARD-TO-FORGET COMMENTS

The negativity you felt from infertility didn't always come just from your own dark thoughts. Without realizing it, those who love and know you best may have hurt you the most with an off-the-cuff remark (or two).

- "When are you going to make me a grandma? I'm tired of waiting!"
- "Why are you so wrapped up in your career? Get going and get pregnant!"
- "You're being a bit self-centered not going to Julie's baby shower, don't you think? It's not her fault you can't get pregnant."
- "Miscarriages are so common, it's nothing to get so upset about. At least you know you can get pregnant."
- "Are you sure you're 'doing it' right? All your sister has to do is look at Mike and boom! she's preggers."
- "It's not like you're going to die. You'll be fine."
- "You can always just adopt. And then you'll probably wind up getting pregnant. That happened to my friend Shirley's daughter's cousin's best friend."

FAMILY TIES

pain and decided to adopt, did your family applaud you? Or did they brazenly give you a hard time, saying you hadn't given enough time or tried hard enough to "have your own"? Were they bothered by your choice to use a surrogate? Are they still trying to understand why you chose the donor egg route?

Whether you felt supported by your family or slightly scarred by their insensitivity, you may wonder if you'll be able to wipe the slate clean once you become a parent.

☞Empty Empathy

I lost my brother—my only brother—when I was pregnant with my son. He died very suddenly. I can honestly say—although hands down, that's the worst experience of my life to date—coping with the infertility was actually harder than coping with the loss of my brother.

When you lose somebody like that, people are really understanding and supportive. They can understand your grief. You're allowed to grieve. I felt like when I was going through the infertility, you get a lot of feelings like somehow you're being selfish by being upset or you know, if you don't want to go to somebody's baby shower, you're the villain. It was really hard.

☞Tracy, 35 (TTC for 3 years; 3-year-old and 7-month-old sons through fertility treatments)

Although they knew you were in terrible emotional pain, your family and friends simply might not have understood it fully, and not have known what you needed. As a matter of fact, maybe you didn't even know what you needed! Was it someone listening mutely to your woes, or someone telling you to buck up? Maybe it changed on an hourly basis. How's that for being impossible?

Your family may have been sympathetic, but what you

really required may have been empathy. For example, you can imagine dealing with a certain diagnosis, ailment, or accident, but until it happens to you, you don't have the same appreciation for it or the capacity to understand the depths and intricacies of feelings it entails. That's why your infertility buddies probably were—and maybe still are—so wonderful. They get it. Your family didn't—at least not fully.

There were words that went unsaid, and hugs that weren't given. Your family wasn't perfect with how they handled your loss. And don't delude yourself: There's always some kind of loss related to infertility. Even though

---

SUPPORT REALLY MATTERS!

Researchers in Germany wanted to find out if social support impacted how well pregnant women fared. They studied 896 women throughout their pregnancies, and found that those with the lowest amount of support from family and friends risked facing the worst outcomes, including having depression and babies with low birth weight. So hug a pregnant or adoption-in-waiting mom today!

---

your infertility has finally been resolved, you can't ignore the fact that you have experienced loss.

There are degrees of loss, of course. Even so, whether you're grieving the fact that your child was conceived in a lab, the babies you lost, or the fact that you'll never have a biological child, infertility always represents something missing to those who have suffered through it.

⌒Reactions to Your Decisions

If there's one thing about infertility, it's that it forces you to be decisive. No matter how long you spent trying to build your family, you faced a series of decisions. You learned that waffling isn't wise. Emotionally, it leaves you unsettled, and financially, it leaves you just as drained. (See Chapter 7, Money Matters.)

If you went through infertility with a significant other, your decisions on next steps were analyzed, probably to death! You had the benefit of mulling things over with someone else. Together you were able to forecast the pros and cons of pursuing a Russian versus a Chinese adoption. You found the calculator to punch out the financial drawbacks of giving IVF "one last try." Maybe your checkbook revealed that giving foster care a try was the most prudent way to go. However the chips landed, you thought it through thoroughly, then acted according to plan. Your decisions were well thought out. Responsible, even!

If you were lucky, your family didn't flinch when you shared your plans with them. While they may have asked questions, they were sensitive ones. They were proud of your maturity, and in your approach to finding a solution. They couldn't wait to be grandparents, no matter how a child came into your life—because it would be your child.

But what if instead of being understanding, your mom and pop flipped out (or worse, weren't the "good kind" of speechless) when you told them which direction you were headed? Did they try to convince you to keep trying, wait to adopt, or campaign hard against adopting from a particular country? Your decisions were questioned to death. Their acceptance didn't come automatically—and maybe they're even still working on it.

If the reactions of your family and friends left something to be desired and you still feel slightly steamed, try to put yourself in their shoes. They didn't have the same access to the rationale behind your family's "master plan" that you did. Remember, you've had time to think things through a lot more than your family. You didn't just wake up one morning and have an epiphany: "Guatemala—of course, that's where we should go to adopt!" You researched it, planned it, and talked to other adoptive parents extensively. Maybe you changed your mind for a time, only to change it right back again.

You don't owe your family and friends the complete, blow-by-blow story, but you should share more information than you would give a total stranger. That info may

MAKE DEFINITIVE—NOT DEBATABLE— DECISIONS

How you deliver a message can be just as important as the message itself. When you state your plans with confidence and conviction, there's less opportunity for anyone to even consider challenging you. For example:

- Instead of, "We're thinking about adopting," Try: "We've contracted an attorney and are going to adopt domestically."
- Instead of, "We might use a donor egg for this round of IVF . . ." Try: "For our final round of IVF we will use a donor egg."
- Instead of, "I'm pregnant with quadruplets," Try: "The doctor recommends that we selectively reduce the pregnancy to twins, to increase our family's chances for a better outcome. We will be following her advice."

hurt—they may need time for their emotions to catch up with the outcome. And it may be difficult for you to put leftover anger or hurt aside, too. Realize that their criticisms weren't directed at you (even if it seemed that way!), but were born out of the frustration of the situation itself. Infertility hurt them, too.

Bottom line: no matter what your level of support was or is today, try not to let it taint your happiness for your new family.

If you've already spilled the beans about your family-building plans, did you waffle or seem unsure about your approach? Maybe now you can understand how the way you shared your news opened your life up to genuinely innocent lines of questioning.

ᗡ Infertility (Part 2)

[After having my first baby] I almost felt like I had a honeymoon from the infertility for a year, where I felt like a normal person, and then the minute I started thinking about having another baby, all those feelings just came back. I wasn't up to snuff, and you know, I would never have a brother or a sister for my son.

You don't really get much support from anybody at that point because they're like, "You have one baby, why are you being selfish?" Almost everyone would say to me, "Do you really have to do that again?" And it was almost like, why do you think I'd want to do this? Like almost as if me having been pregnant "solved" the problem.

ᗡ Tracy, 35 (TTC for 3 years; 3-year-old and
7-month-old sons through infertility treatments)

Will the "real" infertility please stand up?

Primary infertility, or the inability to have your first biological child, is viewed by many as the "real" kind of infer-

102

tility. In addition to your empty heart, you must live in an empty, quiet house.

Secondary infertility, however, can be just as painful and give those who experience it just as much heartache as a first-time-around struggler. (See Chapter 9, Trying Again.) Providing your child with a sibling and simply wanting another baby to love are powerful motivating factors for wanting another child.

It's easy for those on the outside to dismiss secondary infertility as a less serious issue, unfortunately. Many who experience secondary infertility often live in a Catch-22: If people are unaware that you're having trouble conceiving, they think you're selfish for only having one kid; and if they know you'd like to grow your family, they think you're selfish if you're obsessed with trying to conceive. They may even think you're going overboard with treatments if you were able to conceive your first child "naturally."

You know what steps you need to take to build your family. If you choose to, educate your loved ones about your plans. Explain the gory details of what needs to happen. Most likely, they'll soon catch the drift that this certainly isn't your first-choice way of trying to have more children.

If you're going through adoption for the second time around, you may also find that there's less excitement for a second child than there was for the first. Recognize that this happens in "regular" families, too: There's fanfare for the first baby, and subdued celebrations for subsequent ones. Even if you're thrilled to adopt again, it won't be like the first time—after all, you already have a child who takes up much of your time and energy. You're likely to make comparisons, too—if you had a stellar adoption experience the first time, you may worry that you're due for a nightmare

103

FAMILY TIES

this time around. Or if you had a failed placement or waited an extra year, you may dread going through the stress and heartache all over again.

Whether you're adopting or trying to conceive, you shouldn't feel guilty for trying to grow your family. Don't take other people's apathy personally, either. You're the one who's in charge of your family, and you will have the ultimate enthusiasm for who's part of it. (If family members can't understand your efforts, ask them, "How would you feel if my sister didn't exist?" That should provide them with some perspective!)

⌒NATURAL INSTINCTS

[We were already adopting and then found out we were also pregnant.] They were all just beside themselves, ecstatic, happy, except initially my mom, actually. She was much more cautious [saying], "Think about this Suzanne, think about this—where are you going to put two cribs, how are you going to [manage a nine-month-old and a newborn]? You've never been pregnant before . . ."

Ultimately, of course, she came around and shared in the excitement that everybody did. It sticks in my mind even now, and she passed away very unexpectedly two months ago, so you know, now I think of it quite often, and I don't know why I do. I guess it's just those crazy, chaotic days when my two little ones are driving me absolutely up the wall, I wonder, I really wonder if Mom really knew something that I wasn't quite heeding at that moment.

⌒SUZANNE, 38 (TTC FOR 3 YEARS; 9-YEAR-OLD SON THROUGH
DOMESTIC ADOPTION, 5-YEAR-OLD DAUGHTER THROUGH
DOMESTIC ADOPTION, 4-YEAR-OLD "SURPRISE" SON)

As you attempt to repair relationships that were stressed or have gone awry due to infertility, it's important to keep in mind that your family and friends were just looking out for your best interests. While you were all-consumed with becoming a parent, they were biting their nails right along with you. They were also in a better position to forecast what some of the aftershocks of your mission might be. Whether you'd be raising a child with special needs, one who shared only your husband's DNA, or triplets, your family worried about how you were going to manage. And admittedly, if they were parents themselves while you weren't, they probably understood more than you could about the kinds of issues you'd be facing once you became a parent.

You didn't want their worry, of course. You knew the risks and the realities of your own predicament. But you now have the benefit of viewing your painful past through a different lens. Just as you're protective of your child's feelings and future, you realize that your family and friends felt (and hopefully, still feel!) the same way about you. When they saw you in an emotionally vulnerable state, their natural instincts kicked in to high gear to shield you from pain.

> *I'm ashamed of a lot of the feelings that I had when they told us I was pregnant with triplets. I started crying, and it wasn't tears of joy, it was tears of this can't be happening. Both of our moms were pretty happy, I think my husband's dad was pretty happy—but my dad was the worrier. He worried right along with me, he came and stayed with me for a week a couple of months before the babies were due . . . and he told me that he didn't sleep the whole time. He was here and was so worried after he saw how big I was and you know, then*

105

FAMILY TIES

he got worried. They were excited, but they worried right along with us.

—ROBYN, 33 (TTC FOR 3 YEARS; 1-YEAR-OLD TRIPLETS THROUGH FERTILITY TREATMENTS)

Most of the time, comfort came in caring ways.

Your loved ones tracked key dates right along with you, waiting anxiously by their phone or email to hear the latest news. Then they dedicated hours listening to you ramble on about the latest hurdle or crisis, and offered encouraging words or ideas that you maybe hadn't even thought of. They brought you soup and magazines while you were on bed rest, or were recovering from your third D&C. If you were financially stressed, they helped. Money, either in the form of an interest-

You don't choose your family. They are God's gift to you, as you are to them.

—DESMOND TUTU

free loan or with no expectations that it was to be repaid, was a concrete way they showed support for your efforts.

On the flip side, maybe their actions and comments became lost in translation and their instincts to help only managed to hurt. When they criticized the lengthy steps involved in the adoption process, did you take it personally? Did you view open questions about the ethnicity of your yet-to-be-adopted child as snide attacks on him?

Now that you're thankful that your pre-parenting days are over, also be thankful that so many people cared about you during your troubled times—even if the way the care came to you wasn't exactly perfect all of the time (or ever!). Part of what kept you sane during infertility was having support from your family, and they are probably overjoyed at your ultimate success in finally becoming a parent.

ᴄCOMBUSTIBLE REACTIONS

> *When we announced that we were going to adopt from Russia, one of my good friends was very, very negative about our choice. She told me that all of the parents "over there" were drunks, and that all of the children were born with fetal-alcohol syndrome. Her comments were downright hostile.*
>
> ᴄAMY, 44 (TTC FOR 2 YEARS; 3-YEAR-OLD SON AND
> 2-YEAR-OLD DAUGHTER THROUGH INTERNATIONAL ADOPTION)

While it might take more humility than you thought you possessed, you may be able to forgive your family and friends for making caustic comments before they met your child. Naturally, they were curious about your plans, but you now realize they were also worried about you. As you opened their minds to the path you were taking to build your family, though, ideally you also found that you managed to open their hearts.

Hurling ignorant remarks before the child comes on the scene is one thing. But what's impossible to imagine is if these scornful comments are delivered after your child becomes part of your new immediate family. "Zero tolerance" on intolerance is the only stance to take. Your number one priority is your child now, and protecting him from harm is paramount. Verbal abuse, even if it's whispered from behind closed doors, has a way of being heard, and pollutes a person's self-worth more violently than any slap across the face can.

Once your child is part of your life, complete acceptance of him should be expected. If you sense that your family is rejecting your child even in the slightest, you have reason for concern. If you feel inclined to do so (out of earshot of your child, of course), you could confront the offending party. You should hope that they were unaware of their slights—and apologize profusely. If they act blasé, feel pity for them that they're unable to share in the happiness of your new family. Explain your stance, and move on.

More commonly, the rejection isn't overt, but it's still felt. In your heart, you may feel as if your sister's biological kids get more attention from your parents than your adopted ones. You may feel like family members avoid your nine-month-old quadruplets, favoring their easier-to-manage ten-month-old cousin. Unfortunately, playing favorites can happen in even in those "regular" families—and it has absolutely nothing to do with infertility.

If I stop to think before I speak, I won't have to worry afterward about what I said before.

⌐Anonymous

Above everything else, you are the leader of your family and need to decide when you can repair relationships and move onward, or when you need to cut ties. By focusing on

THE BELATED BABY

your own family, you'll experience a sense of freedom and ability to create your own close-knit clan.

Whether your family is traditional-"looking" or as unconventional as they come, your family is legitimate. No one can deny you the right to that legitimacy—and to living without judgment, and in peace.

⌒ Their Point of View on YOU

I guess I'm now just hyper-aware of people's fertility and people's age. I have a sister who just turned thirty, and she's living with a guy and has been with him a long time. I don't think he wants a family and I think she's kind of ambivalent about it, and I just feel like saying, "Look, hon, you're thirty, you don't have that many more years to screw around here."

⌒ JoAnne, 37 (TTC for 4 years; 3-year-old daughter and 5-month-old son through fertility treatments)

After all that you've experienced, there's no doubt that today you are a completely enlightened human being—at least when it comes to family-building issues! You look back now and realize that you might do things differently if you'd known how long it would take you to become a parent. It's too late (and completely unproductive) to lament your own situation, you know—but there's hope for others! You can spread the news! But does your knowledge give you license to warn younger friends about the fragility of their fertility?

Depending on your audience, your message may be appreciated, or rejected with an imperceptible eye roll. Your sister might just want to talk to you about her commitment-phobic boyfriend, and about why he's reluctant about marriage. She isn't ready to even fathom babies yet. Rest assured that if you were open about your fertility, she understands (more than you think she does) that she might face the same troubles herself someday.

Although you want to shout the possible dangers from the rooftops all over town ("Don't wait too long to try!" and "If you're over thirty-five and want children, freeze some eggs today!"), all you might gain is a reputation as a reproduction lunatic. People will start avoiding the topic of babies—or even you—like the plague. Rather than pledge to take an oath of silence on the topic of fertility, listen closely for cues as to when it's appropriate to share your experience. (The answer is often: Never!)

plain worn out

Beyond your tiresome fertility tooting, others in the family may have grown worn out by being immersed alongside you in your saga. (Hey, give them a break—you were sick of it, too!) They endured your mood swings and repeated disappointments. Their ears grew hot pressing the phone receiver against their head, listening to your lengthy, gloomy tales. To bring over flowers or a home-cooked meal to you, they shifted their own schedules to give you some much-needed TLC.

And how did you repay them at the time? Often, with your absence.

Maybe your best friend was deeply hurt that you couldn't muster up the strength to go to her baby's christening. Or you missed an out-of-state wedding because you had an appointment for an egg retrieval. You and your partner skipped Christmas because you just couldn't bear to be around all of the nieces and nephews who would be there. In the end, your troubles garnered more of the family's attention and as a result, attention was taken away from special occasions. Even though you believed that life was just carrying on without you, you now realize that you may

110

have inadvertently disappointed a few folks along the way.

Of course, a new child has a way of overshadowing past indiscretions and bringing everyone together. Your joy is their joy, and chances are that the celebrations for your new child will outshine and outlast the dark times. While there's no reason to feel guilty, it's also never wrong to notice and remember the sacrifices that your loved ones made for you. A handwritten note that simply states the fact that you love someone and appreciate how they cared for you can go a long way in multiplying the joy of your new child.

⌒Building Family Character

Infertility reveals the dark side of everything. Not having a child the way nature intended causes loneliness, anger, and anxiety—not just for you and your partner, but for everyone who knows and loves you best. Although they weren't perfect in showing total support to you, you weren't perfect, either.

When you set aside the past feelings of guilt and frustration permanently, you can celebrate the fact that it helped your family grow closer together. The people who love you witnessed your turmoil and shared in your ups and downs—even if they didn't say so. You're now an "infertility survivor," and so is your entire family.

Just as you can look back now and testify to the ways infertility strengthened your marriage, you can also see how it deepened your relationship with others who love you— or at least made you appreciate the unique bonds of family. That can be another "gift" of infertility.

6

Bitterness Isn't Beautiful:
YOUR RELATIONSHIP WITH OTHER PARENTS
(AND THE WORLD)

[Infertility] impacts me every day and I hate that it does. But if I'm honest with myself, I know that it does. If I hear someone's pregnant, my first thought still is, I'll bet you didn't work as hard as I did. Or, how come you got pregnant, but my friend Darlene who's been trying for nine years and is the nicest person I know still isn't pregnant? I'm not even to the point yet where my first thought is "congratulations." It's still, "Hmmm, well, I'll bet you just got drunk and got pregnant."

⌐AMANDA, AGE 36 (TTC FOR 5 YEARS; 3-YEAR-OLD AND
1-YEAR-OLD DAUGHTERS THROUGH FERTILITY TREATMENTS)

When you're in the heat of infertility, it consumes your entire life.

Your work plays second fiddle to your lineup of monthly treatments. Ovulation waits for no one and nothing. That inane conference call or business trip overseas must be postponed on the whim that this will be the time it works. Your life is constantly imposed upon by either fertilizing or getting fertilized, and you're discouraged by having to impose your ridiculous schedule upon others.

Your social life also suffers. If you know other parents,

especially new parents, you know how it seems that conversation always turns back to kids, whether you're at a cocktail party, a barbeque, a dinner out, or a neighborhood get-together. Maybe the people you met knew you were "trying," and maybe they didn't. But chances are that you started turning down invites, either because you weren't up to acting happy, didn't want to be asked about when you'd be having a baby, or a combination of both.

Worst of all? The dreaded baby shower invitation. (That tenth friend in a row just announced her pregnancy!) You either grinned and showed up with booties and a blanket or dodged the gathering entirely to protect your heart, just a little, from yet another celebration that wouldn't be yours.

Month after month, year after year, the hectic schedule and perpetual disappointment added to your resentment— toward your body, the situation, and the world.

But wait! You've finally succeeded! You're a parent, or will be one soon. It's your day to shine. So why do you occasionally feel the same resentment that you did during your pre-kid days?

When you've gone through so much angst, hardship, and heartaches, it can be hard to just "forget about it" and move on. Whether it's feeling jealous toward a pregnant person or believing that a fellow parent who is surrounded by kids doesn't fully appreciate her good fortune, you might be surprised when those old infertility feelings surface. You may even feel a tad superior (or a lot superior) to other parents because you went through hell to have your child. The resentment that built up during the infertile years may not automatically evaporate and can manifest in different ways. By dealing with leftover infertile emotions, you can move on to create meaningful relationships with fellow parents, regardless of how they got there.

114

⌒FRIENDSHIPS AFTER INFERTILITY

When you were hoping to become a parent, maybe you glamorized the other side of the fence. Once you were a mom yourself, you imagined, you'd immediately fall into a close circle of fellow moms, and find all the love and laughter and support they seemed to share when you were watching from "outside." You'd no longer feel alone, or outside the group—with a baby, you've gained entrée, at last!

If only it were that easy. Friendships can be just as challenging once you become a parent as they were before—or at least as complex. One of the best ways to work through your residual bitter feelings is by having strong, supportive friendships. But after going through infertility, those friendships may have changed.

through thick and thin

Did you reach out to your friends during your fertility struggles, or retreat and become a total recluse? How you went about managing your social life during your darkest days may influence who your best buddies will be as you enter parenthood.

If you are the type of person who talks openly and often about all aspects of your life, you probably wore your heart on your sleeve pre-kid. Many of your friends may have known month-by-month (or day-by-day) what you were experiencing, and followed your cycles right along with you like watching a real-life soap opera. They sent cards and candy after each failed attempt, and backed you 100 percent when you vowed to try again.

If a friend had gone through infertility herself, she may have been extra tuned in to your needs, and perfectly understanding about your moods. She didn't require a lengthy explanation of each procedure; she didn't judge you on the ethics of your choices. If she was green about what is involved in treatments, though, you grew to dread her looks of pity, especially if she was busy managing a crew of kids herself.

In either case, your friendships either grew stronger, or eventually your woes wore out their welcome. Infertility served as a litmus test, and filtered out the true friends from the flakes. You emerged from the experience knowing who will stand by you and help you now to become the best parent you can be.

fellow infertile friends

[Before getting pregnant], I used to think getting pregnant and continuing to be part of my infertility support group would actually give the group hope. However, it's not a good place to be when you're pregnant. I just put myself in their shoes. It's so depressing to be in that room, and usually the meetings last two hours. There are horror stories. People have given up hope, and just have never gotten pregnant. I don't know. I kind of feel guilty.

⌒ASHLEY, 34 (TTC FOR 2 YEARS; PREGNANT WITH FIRST CHILD THROUGH FERTILITY TREATMENTS)

You're fortunate if you've maintained friends throughout infertility and parenthood. But if you expanded your circles and created a new set of friends in the infertility underground, you may find yourself estranged from these people once you become a parent.

After all, you remember how it felt when another person who was in the trenches of infertility announced her success. Although you were happy for each victor and knew intellectually that it had nothing to do with you, emotionally it felt like a dagger through your own heart that you weren't the pregnant one. You remember a subdued and sheepish "I'm pregnant, guys" or the online subject line header "BFP++++++++" from a fellow infertile. You were politely enthusiastic when someone was exiting the process, but you'd always thought that you were next.

When it is finally your turn to be the lucky one, you're elated, but you're also sensitive and want more than anything not to sting others with your news of becoming a parent. You may feel guilty, as if you are betraying your friends. You want to give them hope and not discourage them from continuing to pursue being a parent, but it might be impossible to disguise the fact that you are one.

Continuing to relate with certain groups can pose a Catch-22. You don't want to preach from the pulpit of parenthood, but you also may feel wiser than you were during treatments. For example, if someone is jamming five embryos into her uterus during IVF, you're in a more comfortable—and therefore rational—position than she is to see the danger in her decision. If you adopted, you may want to spread the word that this is best way to resolve infertility of all—why continue to torture your body when there are babies to be had elsewhere? You feel caught in the middle.

Just remember that everyone has her own destiny to play out, and the true friends are the ones who will stick by you and share in your successes and failures—and you for them. Surface friends come together because they share a particular time in life, and infertility can be one of those times. While you may miss the camaraderie of those friends, it was probably rooted in the drama of infertility. Now you have the drama of parenting ahead of you, and you'll have the chance to connect with plenty of new friends who are parenting kids the same age as yours.

BITTERNESS ISN'T BEAUTIFUL

always different

> When my daughter was born, I felt like a fish out of water. At forty years old and inexperienced, I wasn't sure how to act with a baby. I remember going to the mall when she was three weeks old and she was in her stroller and I saw other moms with strollers and I felt like a fraud, like I didn't belong with them.
>
> ⌐KIM, 44 (TTC FOR 5 YEARS; 4-YEAR-OLD DAUGHTER THROUGH FERTILITY TREATMENTS AND GESTATIONAL SURROGATE)

> I signed up for a "Mommy and Me" class, but it wasn't for me. I didn't feel like I bonded with the mothers at all. I didn't feel like I fit in . . . I felt like I was old. And I think in the end, I realized that it wasn't that I thought I was old, or that I was so much older than them, but I had such a different experience than all of them: Their children came so easily, and I just could not relate to them.
>
> One of them I remember was saying how—we were talking about how having children has changed the way we conduct our lives, you know, how you can't do everything for yourself, you're not first anymore. You can't go out when you want, you can't do whatever you want anymore, and one girl said, "My baby hasn't cramped my style! I'm still a party girl, we still go out, I just take her wherever I go with me, she's great, we go out to lunch, we go out to parties."
>
> She was very defensive. I just thought, my children have *changed* my life—that's the point! I do everything for them! I don't just drag them along with me everywhere, I do what's in their best interest. I don't know, I just was kind of, some of the moms were like, oh, this baby is weighing me down.
>
> ⌐LISA, 33 (TTC FOR 2 YEARS; NEWBORN BOY/GIRL TWINS THROUGH FERTILITY TREATMENTS)

THE BELATED BABY

Your past may give you a unique perspective that will also influence who you're inclined to befriend in the future. If there's a group that laughs knowingly that their husbands just look at them and "poof!" they're pregnant, for example, you might find you have less in common with them since their experience was so different from your own. That's not to insinuate that you don't or won't have friends who are fabulously fertile, because you will. It's just that it might be harder to fully connect with someone who never had first-hand experience with infertility, and who doesn't understand how the anguish you felt stays with you and changes you.

Accept the fact that you'll never feel like a "regular" parent, because you *aren't* a regular parent. You'll never know what it's like to have babies on demand. You had to work harder to get to the parenting starting gate than most of the people around you, and you had to put your life on hold.

There are few experiences more intense than infertility, and going through it can sometimes make you prematurely mature. From the lessons of infertility, you've gained patience, determination, and self-control. Fortunately, these stellar qualities are quite useful when it comes to parenting, too!

branching out

It was hard when [my child] was . . . one or two years old and I would go to those "Mommy, Baby, Music" classes and everyone would say "Oh, I'm pregnant again" or "Oh, I'm having my third." And they would go on and on and on . . . after I'd just had a miscarriage.

That was very isolating, because though I was not without child, I was never going to be one of them. And it's kind of that way now, even as my child is older. I'm never really going to be one of them because they complain, "Oh, I've got too many kids, the kids are driving

119

me crazy, the house is a mess." And they complain about the kids all the time.

⌐MARGARET, 47 (TTC FOR 6 YEARS; 9-YEAR-OLD SON
THROUGH FERTILITY TREATMENTS)

Parenting—or least parenting well—is one of the hardest jobs in the world. It's a physically and mentally demanding role, and one that nothing can truly prepare you for. On top of it all, the pay is downright horrible.

So what gets you through another day of it? Friends, of course!

You can find almost any virtual buddy who fits your same profile and circumstance. Many fertility websites have "parenting after infertility" message boards (e.g., www.theafa.org, www.resolve.org, and www.inciid.org), and you can hook up with fellow parents with kids the same as age as yours. If you want to distance yourself from the infertile set, try www.ivillage.com, www.family.com, www.babble.com/babblepedia, www.momspace.com, and www.mops.org. Some of the sites have bulletin boards, and others have "collaborative" features where you can swap your best parenting secrets with other parents.

Of course, nothing can replace an IRL (in real life), face-to-face friend. During the tot gym class or preschool sing-a-long, try to bask in the moments that make up your life today instead of grumbling about the thoughtless (though usually not malicious) comments from the fertile Myrtles. Look for another parent or two you connect with—they are out there! Here's the thing—you won't like every parent. You won't bond with every other fellow mother. In fact, you'll find that you can't stand some of them! But that doesn't mean you won't make friends.

Immerse yourself in the world of your two-year-old and reach out to other moms with two-year-olds to commiserate about how terrible—and also terrific—this stage can be. While you might not share a common conception history with these other moms and dads, a two-year-old has a way of bringing you immediately into the moment. The more you connect with other parents about the experiences you're sharing now, the less alienated you will feel about the things that make you different from the rest—and the more likely you will be to find like-minded friends.

Finally, be gentle, not judgmental, with others who seem cavalier when it comes to having children. Think of it this way: You've had more time to adjust to the thought of being a parent than someone who simply decided to become pregnant and then did. In preparation for the role of parent, you prepared your mind as well as your house, job, and priorities. You've been ready to enter the role for a long time, and in many ways are more ready for the responsibility. It's okay to feel a little smug sometimes. Just don't wallow in it.

⌐The "Obvious" Infertile

I don't think I look my age, but I certainly don't look thirty. I don't think I look fifty. I think I look maybe in my early forties. Even so, I've been asked if I was a grandmother.

⌐Rebecca, 50 (TTC for 4 years; 4-year-old boy/girl twins through fertility treatments and donor egg)

Remember, even if a woman looks like she has it all—handsome, attentive husband; beautiful, easily conceived children; meaningful work; drop-dead looks; and abs you can bounce a quarter off of—you have no way of knowing what she's been through. Maybe she had multiple miscarriages. Maybe her husband just admitted he's having an affair. Maybe they're about to lose that beautiful house you

121

BITTERNESS ISN'T BEAUTIFUL

envy. You can't tell everything about someone just by looking at him or her.

The same is true of you, too. Maybe no one can tell by looking at you how you suffered to be a parent, or that you still deal with leftover emotions today. But while people can't know about everything, what if they can "tell" about your infertility? What if you're an "obvious infertile," or someone who looks different from the parental "norm"? Maybe you have twins after the age of forty, you're parenting an only child when everyone around you has two or three, or your kids look different from you. People demand an explanation. Suddenly everyone wants to know how you became a parent, why you don't have another child, or where all of those kids came from. You feel as if you've been transported from the fertility doctor's waiting room to the freak show stage at the circus!

The comments from people will range from amusing to downright rude, causing you to wonder how many people were raised in a barn. If you were somehow cajoled into

COMMENTS TO EXPECT WHEN YOU ADOPT

"Where'd you get him from?"
"He is so lucky you adopted him."
"Why would anyone give up such a beautiful child?"
"Aren't you afraid they're going to take him back?"
"Do you know his real parents?"
"How much did you pay for him?"
"Why didn't you have your own?"
"Do you have any real kids?"
"Does she speak Chinese?" (about a Chinese-ancestry toddler with Caucasian parents)

THE BELATED BABY

COMMENTS TO EXPECT WHEN YOU HAVE MULTIPLES

"Are they all yours?"

"You poor thing."

"I would kill myself."

"Can you tell them apart?"

"Did you want this many kids?"

"Did you have to 'do it' three times to get triplets?" (Commentator then laughs with great hilarity at the "originality" of his comment.)

"Did you go through fertility treatments?"

"How much did those kids cost?"

disclosing the fact that you used fertility drugs, be prepared to field extensive comments about the process. The topic of your sex life is also free game. Whether infinitely curious or exceptionally stupid, the public will request information from you that's not always (or ever!) their right to know.

The barrage of comments you receive when you're out and about as a family can be a constant reminder of the reason why your family is the way it is: Infertility. Maybe your child is Chinese and you're Caucasian. If you're an older parent, people may assume that your child is adopted or you used donor sperm or egg—if they don't first think that you're a grandparent. Have twins or more? The chance of having multiples increases by 20 to 25 percent if you've used reproductive technologies.

⌒DEALING WITH THE IGNORANT . . . AND THE MEAN

If you're asked personal questions, the good news is that you can choose to share only if you wish—or decide not to at all.

COMMENTS TO EXPECT WHEN YOU'RE AN OLDER PARENT

"Is he yours?"

"Was he a surprise?"

"You're such an involved grandparent."

"Does he wear you out?"

"You poor thing."

"Did you go through fertility treatments?"

"Here you go—hand this to your grandma!" (Said to the child.)

While some comments you'll field will be undoubtedly silly, others can downright sting. Derogatory remarks about how you conceived your children or adoption in general can throw you into a tizzy about your abilities as a parent. If you're self-conscious about how you became a parent, you might be particularly vulnerable to feeling defensive or ashamed of your story.

When someone says something that seems hateful, rewind and replay the comment in your mind before you respond. Most likely, your mood will determine if you respond negatively or humorously. Above all else, try not to take it personally. Imagine all of the people who are on your side and support you and how you created your family, which will give you a positive outlook about how to answer.

The more questions you answer about your family and fertility, the more you realize that (most) people have good hearts and wholesome intentions. People don't understand reproductive technologies as much as you do—and ignorance is their bliss. They also don't think before they speak,

You'll hear plenty of silly, nosy, and downright rude questions as an "obvious" infertile. Anticipate the questions that will be asked of you, and have your arsenal of answers at the ready. A few ideas for responding to the clueless include:

- "I'm sorry, do I know you?"
- "Wow! That's a personal question, isn't it?"
- "Why do you ask?"

and often feel remorse as soon as the words escape from their big mouths. You'll probably find that many people who are curious about your past are so because they are worried about their own fertility or have a family member who has just embarked down the road for reproductive help. Be sensitive to them (which will inspire them to reciprocate some sensitivity toward you!).

As your children grow, you'll need to include them in your practice sessions of how to respond to those who ask about your family's history. (See Chapter 8, Your Family's Story.) Remember, your child watches you at all times, and your positive interactions will go far in how he views the world. If you try to approach each interaction with humor and kindness, you'll help leave those bitter feelings behind—and set the stage for raising happy, secure children as well.

spontaneous vs. simulated multiples

People always ask me when they see the twins, "Oh, does it run in your family?" And I never know how to respond! It actually does run in my family and my husband's family, so I just respond, "Yes." But I feel like it's

125

a lie, like I'm not telling a lie, but I'm not giving the whole truth. But I don't know these people! They're strangers! Still, it's always a little odd and it makes me feel a little strange. And then it's always kind of strange if I'm with someone who knows they're IVF babies.

⌒MARISA, 37 (TTC FOR 4 YEARS; 2-YEAR-OLD BOY/GIRL TWINS THROUGH FERTILITY TREATMENTS)

Having "natural" or spontaneous twins (or those conceived without the help of fertility treatments) is rare. The odds of having "natural" fraternal twins is only 1 in 60, and the odds of identical twins is even rarer, 1 in 250. Thanks to fertility drugs and delayed childbirth, though, we're surrounded by more manufactured multiples than ever before. According to the National Center for Health Statistics, between 1980 and 2000 the number of twin births has increased 74 percent and the number of higher order multiples (triplets or more) increased fivefold. That means that about 3 percent of babies in the United States are born in sets of two, three, or more, and about 95 percent of these multiple births are twins.

You might feel as if you're living a lie when people ask you about the origins of your brood, since you have a set of these "unnatural" kids on your hands. You might feel as if your twins aren't as genuine as the real deal, even though you're just as much up to your elbows in diapers as that mom who conceived twins the old-fashioned way!

In fact, a definite dynamic exists between parents of multiples who were created spontaneously and those who created theirs back at the lab. You may run into fellow twin parents, for instance, who repeatedly claim that twins "run in their family." (That's your hint that their children are of the natural variety.) You might wonder if there's an unspoken caste system—and that you're at the bottom of it!

126

You might also feel an overwhelming sense of guilt for creating multiples via reproductive technologies when asked about your kids. You may feel like a fraud, for example, when people ask if your kids have a certain secret "twin" language or other identical twin phenomena. What applies solely to studies of identical twins (which are more common with spontaneous conception) has no relevance to your fraternal twins who were more "ART-fully" conceived. When senior citizens stop you in the mall to marvel at your triplets since it's such a rarity to them (the odds of having them "naturally" is only 1 of 8,100), you might feel sheepish about their attention. They are unaware that the National Center for Health Statistics found that from 1980 to 1997, the triplet and higher order birth rate increased 400 percent—and 1,000 percent for women in their forties.

No one can make you feel inferior without your permission.

⌒Eleanor Roosevelt
(1884–1963)

Your odds were upped, and now you're the one who feels odd! But when people stop and drill you with questions, understand that people love to see children and are curious about how you manage your day more than how you conceived your kids. If someone acts like she's superior to you with her identical twins in tow, maybe that's the only accomplishment she's ever had in her life. Pity her, not yourself!

⌒Know Your Limits

Now that you're a parent, your infertility no longer consumes you. You've accepted the fact that things didn't go smoothly for you in building your family. Maybe you wouldn't change a thing about your family today. But you may still need to protect yourself from certain situations if they are painful.

127

Just because you're a full-fledged parent doesn't mean that cuddling another woman's infant will hold instant appeal for you, for instance. In addition to the baby, wrapped in that blanket might be a bundle of your unresolved emotions, and holding it may bring on an acute sense of regret and loss for what might have been. For example, if you're worried about your next round of treatments to create a new brother or sister for your child, your secondary infertility may make it painful to even catch a whiff of someone else's infant.

If you are surrounded by multiples, you might feel angry that you weren't able to lavish attention on each one of your children when they were newborns—so why should you do the same for someone else's baby now? If you adopted an older child, being around an infant might make your heart ache for the fact that you weren't able to hold your child at that exact age and take care of her from the very start of her life. If your baby was colicky or you experienced post-partum depression or general feelings of inadequacy, you might feel as if you were robbed of the chance to enjoy babyhood. Being around other people's babies brings it all back.

Face it: Every baby you meet and greet from now on will represent something more than just a milk-guzzling, pooping machine. You will relate each small person back to your own situation, and you might continue to feel pangs of jealousy. If you're unable to stomach attending a baby shower or feel uneasy about visiting the infant of an acquaintance, don't feel guilty for taking a pass . . . at least this time.

⌒COMPLAINTS ABOUT COMPLAINERS

In the beginning when the babies were little, I would go to these [twins group] meetings and I found that it was

THE BELATED BABY

one big bitch session. These women were complaining about how much work it was having multiples, and I could not stand it. I wanted to just jump up and say, "Oh my God, I absolutely adore having these babies!" When they were infants, I was the happiest, most joyful mom you've ever seen.

‟ANITA, 43 (TTC FOR 4 YEARS; 7-YEAR-OLD TWIN SONS
THROUGH FERTILITY TREATMENTS AND DONOR EGG)

When you're a new parent, it's likely that you're stressed out somehow. Whether you're completely sleep-deprived, dealing with your child's or your own health issues, or are immersed in nailing the bonding process, you've certainly earned the right to moan and whine, at least a little bit. Even so, you probably feel more obliged than most—and also more obligated—to keep your chin up and smile. This is everything you've ever wanted, so you must behave accordingly and act extra grateful at all times for being so blessed, right? (See Chapter 3, Parents at Last.)

You might believe (or know) that people who didn't work as hard as you did to become parents consider parent-hood to be a complete pain in the rear. For them, just having a kid has given them a permanent license to complain. Their litany of woes might include the high cost of diapers, how demanding it is to juggle a career and childcare, and how sick they are of wearing clothes stained with spit-up. (The list could continue endlessly, as every parent knows.)

Your tolerance for their grumbles might be zero. You empathize, but you also know how lucky you are to be enjoying the experience of parenthood. While you'll proba-bly spend your time with parents who are as level-headed as you are, you're also bound to cross paths with at least a few of the martyrs. Instead of feeling frustrated or avoiding certain people entirely, try to understand their points of

129

view. Did they become pregnant accidentally and now are unprepared for reality of raising kids? Do they come from an unstable home life themselves, and so are unsure of their ability to parent?

Listen to their stories—both good and bad—and be willing to share a few of your own, too. By sharing the ups and downs of your infertility struggle, you might shed some light on why you appreciate parenthood so much, which might be contagious! People who considered childbirth to be an invasive and disruptive part of their lives might benefit from hearing about your laparoscopy, repeated vaginal ultrasounds, or seven miscarriages followed by D&Cs. By hearing your history, others might take their parenthood a little less for granted.

⌒SPOKESPERSON SYNDROME

It's funny, my friends call me the "fertility guru," because I have random people calling me—like, friends of friends or acquaintances will be like, "Can I talk to you about [fill in the fertility topic]?" And I'm like the fertility sergeant. I just try to educate them.

⌒TRACY, 35 (TTC FOR 3 YEARS; 3-YEAR-OLD AND 7-MONTH-OLD SONS THROUGH FERTILITY TREATMENTS)

There's another side to surviving infertility. You are now one of the more enlightened people in town when it comes to building a family. You know there aren't any guarantees and that just because you go off the pill in September doesn't mean a bundle of joy is on its way in June. You take pity on the naive, and your informed point of view may cause you to be a mouthpiece (or loudmouth) when it comes to dealing with other people's fertility. Whether you wanted to or not, you may find that you've taken on the role of fertility consultant to both friends and strangers.

130

Be judicious in how you use your knowledge, though. If you're the type who just can't bite her tongue and you meet with your city friend who's thirty-nine and still hasn't connected with Mr. Right, your "advice" that she freeze some eggs as soon as she has some free time might sound harsh. Listen patiently, and the opportunity to advise will arise. If a friend seems receptive to ideas or wants your opinion, share your story.

When people seek your opinion, you can be of great service to them. As you may have experienced, an in-person meeting with someone who's been there/done that can go far in improving someone else's experience with infertility treatments. Whether it's recommending a course of treatment or connecting with a specific doctor who specializes in recurring miscarriages, you appreciated the care someone showed to you by providing their input. If you knew of someone who was successful in transitioning from treatment to adoption, you gained strength from their counsel.

Now that you're a parent, you probably feel obligated to pass it on and to help others in their time of crisis. If you're part of a formal fertility organization, you may have success in reaching out to those who are receptive to your message. Your experience allows you to find the right words to reach those who are in despair; you know how they feel and can guide them through.

With your new parental perspective, you may find it draining to hear the sad stories of infertility. You may relive painful memories that you'd rather keep in the past. If you find this is the case, keep your past separate from your current life. While you don't need to abandon your personal history and ability to guide others altogether, don't turn it into your life. Save some of that energy for your family and children.

131

You believe what people tell you about how you can get pregnant until you're forty, don't worry about it. But you know, you don't really know the truth of what people go through. You see all these Hollywood stars having babies at forty-four and forty-five, and I know that they're donor egg babies. But I didn't know it [before I went through infertility], you know? People don't disclose that sort of thing. I think you should be upfront about it. I think if more people were upfront about it, people would understand that the clock is ticking.

⌒MARGARET, 47 (TTC FOR 6 YEARS; 9-YEAR-OLD SON
THROUGH FERTILITY TREATMENTS)

When I was forty-five, people would look at me and see an older mom with infants. Then they read People *magazine and they look at Joan Lunden, who used a surrogate, and think that's normal. But she never says anything about those eggs. She never admits to not using her eggs.*

⌒REBECCA, 50 (TTC FOR 4 YEARS; 4-YEAR-OLD BOY/GIRL
TWINS THROUGH FERTILITY TREATMENTS AND DONOR EGG)

A quick flip through any tabloid magazine will cause you to doubt that a woman's fertility declines after age thitry-five. In fact, it may even cause someone to believe that it actually increases after that age!

Like disguising plastic surgeries or eating disorders, many stars seem unwilling to come clean about the truth behind their feats with fertility. (For example, is Joan Lunden biologically related to her twins? Does it matter?) Unfortunately, the lack of openness from some might have the negative effect of perpetuating the myth that getting pregnant can magically happen at any age.

132

While you might resent the lack of total honesty, consider the fact that those who are in the public eye deserve privacy. Behind the glitz and glamour might be their pain of using donor eggs or going through IVF. No one can relate better than you—a fellow former infertile!

ᴄ̄Let Go of What Wasn't

My sister was seven months pregnant with her fourth and giving me a tour of the nursery. It was all ready to go, with fresh paint, new bedding, and a closet filled with tiny pink dresses on tiny pink hangers. I was overcome with envy, feeling regret that I never had the chance to savor my own pregnancy and properly prepare. With all of the doctor appointments, weight gain and worry that everyone would be born fine, being pregnant with triplets isn't something you savor.

ᴄ̄Jill, 38 (TTC for 3 years; 7-year-old girl/boy/boy triplets through fertility treatments)

Here's some old news: Infertility treatments aren't part of anyone's ideal way to build a family. Whether your need for fertility help was due to medical problems, age, or the aggravating "unexplained" diagnosis, there are few people who are pleased to grace the entrance of a fertility clinic. Even if you sidestepped the treatment route entirely and headed straight for growing your family through adoption, you may have encountered twinges of remorse along the way that this was your fate.

If you suffered through multiple miscarriages, you've felt the heartache of a missed opportunity and grieved the loss of your child. Through the months and years ahead, you may continue to remember each miscarriage and reflect wistfully as each due date comes and goes. You may wonder about the person who could have been, especially when you see chil-

133

dren the same age running around as your still-missed children. It might be hard to maintain friendships with people who have older children, especially since their little league schedule doesn't ever mesh with your child's nap times.

If you haven't already done so, acknowledge your lost fantasy and accept the fact that your experience wasn't ideal or the one that you had imagined. Then remind yourself that no one's truly is. (After all, even that woman who's got it made in the fertility shade probably has obstacles and troubles in other areas of her life.)

As an infertility survivor, you know better than most people how little control we have over our lives. After you acknowledge the loss of your "dream family," embrace the reality and love the people who are your family today.

◌PERSONALITY IMPROVEMENTS (COMPLIMENTS OF INFERTILITY?)

I think [infertility] has allowed me to give more people the benefit of the doubt. I used to sit there, and even if somebody was pregnant, I would . . . as a non-pregnant person, I would think, "Oh, I'm sure your life was so easy, you have no idea what I'm going through." And I finally got to the spot where I figured out, you know, she may have had exactly the same problem I did. And I just don't know it, I'm just seeing the end product. So, I try and remember that in pretty much all my dealings with everybody. I like to think of myself as enlightened, but that moment where I realize, "Oh, you know what, they may have had just the same kind of problems I did." I guess at the end of the day I can say it's made me a better person.

◌AMANDA, 36 (TTC FOR 5 YEARS; 3-YEAR-OLD AND
1-YEAR-OLD DAUGHTERS THROUGH FERTILITY TREATMENTS)

For a while, even after my older daughter was born, I still kind of felt like I was part of the infertile world I think a little bit, maybe it was just because it was fresh in my mind, or maybe it was because, you know, I knew I wouldn't be able to conceive a second so easily. But now that I have two, I definitely am not feeling like I'm in that world anymore—it's becoming more of a distant memory, let's say. But I don't know if it's just because of time, or because I have two.

—JOANNE, 37 (TTC FOR 4 YEARS; 3-YEAR-OLD DAUGHTER AND
5-MONTH-OLD SON THROUGH FERTILITY TREATMENTS)

There are a host of reasons to be bitter about how rocky your road was in becoming a parent. It's not fair that you couldn't have a baby right when you wanted one. It's not fair that you had to travel to a faraway country to find your child. It's not fair that you've missed out on childbirth, and then you have to hear all about what it's like from your new parental peers. It's all just, well, NOT FAIR!

To repeat what your mother probably told you, "Life's not fair!"

But if you look past your anger, you'll see that infertility has residual benefits. First of all, you have more appreciation for the wonder of your child (or children) and for being a parent. Because you know better than anyone that things don't always work out the way you'd wanted them to, you're probably more in tune with other people's needs and sympathetic about their problems than you were before infertility. That's one of the gifts you've received, whether you asked for it or not. Your compassion—compliments of infertility—is strong, and will allow you to move past your resentment and have a positive outlook on life.

BITTERNESS ISN'T BEAUTIFUL

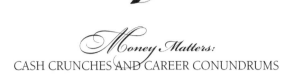

7

Money Matters:
CASH CRUNCHES AND CAREER CONUNDRUMS

When we started with the adoption process, I was a little unsure because there was no guarantee that it was going to happen. I wondered, will adopting take six months? Eight months? A year? It was also very expensive, and we were coming off of infertility treatments and owed thousands of dollars for that. (We'd found out that our insurance company wouldn't pay for our last procedures, and then they refused to cover us at all.) I was looking at the business end of it—adoption is very expensive—and I thought, "Is this even going to happen?" I definitely had some anxiety about the money involved. I hated to break it down to dollars and cents, but that's how I'm wired.

⌒GARY, 44 (TTC 13 YEARS, 7-YEAR-OLD
THROUGH DOMESTIC ADOPTION)

How much would you spend to keep your belated baby in your life?

Cruel question with an obvious answer: You'd spend everything you have, own, and will ever earn—and then a million times over again—to keep your kid around. Your child is your most prized possession—she is priceless.

137

So then, how much did it cost to bring her into your life?

When you go through infertility it's a black-and-white fact that the expense far exceeded how much a "natural kid" would have set you back, and more than you had originally expected—or budgeted for!

You have experienced firsthand that infertility treatments not only take time, but also money . . . sometimes a lot of it. From costly procedures and drugs to adoption agency fees and plane tickets, your baby bills started coming due long before (and sometimes long after) there was ever a known due date for delivery marked down on your calendar.

Raising a child is expensive, but for people with infertility, simply getting that child in the first place can cost tens of thousands of dollars. Your obligations came not only in the form of dollars, but also in personal sacrifice. Instead of a vacation or a fancy car, you plunked down cash for a sperm washing (and other procedures you had no idea even existed before your troubles started). And once you ran out of your own funds, you either had to take a second job, max out a few credit cards, or swallow your pride and ask family members for money to avoid going into debt.

If insurance didn't pick up at least part of the tab, maybe debt was unavoidable and you still have bills left over from infertility treatment. As a result, credit cards, second mortgages, or other loans might have been your only avenue to pay for adoption expenses. Whether you're free from debt or facing a mountain of it, there's been a price tag associated with your belated baby, one that other parents can't even fathom.

Now that you have an amazingly expensive baby on your hands, you're dealing with a whole new set of financial

138

COMPARING BABY-MAKIN' BUDGETS

Budget to **Make** *a Baby ("naturally"):*

1. Selecting a fine wine and getting busy in bed a night (or two, just to be sure—wink, wink) ($24)
2. Cavalierly picking up a generic one-pack home pregnancy test at the drug store just to confirm that the twinge you felt was, in fact, implantation ($10)
3. Knowing that you're with the child who was meant for you, and you were meant for him: Priceless

Budget to **Fake** *a Baby (with a doctor's assistance):*

1. Buying wine once, then predicting and scrutinizing when ovulation occurs and having missionary-style sex followed by legs high up in the air over 250 mornings, noons, and nights ($24 for the first bottle of wine, which eventually becomes water)
2. Forking over $865 for an IUI, $8,158 for each IVF, and, since you're a go-getter, $1,544 for an intracytoplasmic sperm injection (ICSI) and $3,550 for a PGD. And wait! Don't forget the extra $3,000 to $5,000 needed for IVF medications.* Oh, and another $10,000 (or more) if using donor eggs
3. Knowing that you're with the child who was meant for you, and you were meant for him: Priceless

(*Average costs provided from RESOLVE, based on a cross-section of clinics willing to share the info; not surprisingly, not all were willing to do so.)

Budget to **Take** *a Baby (adoption):*

1. Buying wine to cheer that treatment is over (or never even started in the first place) ($24)
2. Signing up with an adoption agency or attorney, if private adoption ($1,500)
3. Paying fees for domestic adoption ($5,000 to $40,000—or more) or international adoption ($7,000 to $30,000)
4. Knowing that you're with the child who was meant for you, and you were meant for him: Priceless.

pressures—and a new sense of guilt if you make the "wrong" decision. Should you or your spouse stay home to be a full-time parent? Are you willing to put your career on hold, or leave it behind indefinitely? If you were blessed with "extra" kids (you had multiples), you may find yourself in a Catch-22: you can't afford not to work, but you can't afford daycare for your quads, either.

If you decide that both you and your spouse must work, can you withstand the judgment that might come your way from others?

Anticipating and managing the financial needs of a family can be tricky. What's trickier, still, is affording a kid if you're in a financial hole from the start.

I feel really guilty, because my husband is perfect, and I feel guilty that he works so hard and a lot of our procedures weren't covered. We've spent thousands of dollars on healthcare related issues because of infertility. You know, we can't get a new car and we can't go on vacation, and I'm frustrated. The government goes on and on about family values, yet they won't help pay to create a family. They'll pay for an eighty-year-old's Viagra, but they won't pay for my fertility meds so I can have a child. So it's frustrating, but we're very lucky. My parents have been incredibly supportive.

CJENNIFER, 37 (TTC FOR 3 YEARS; 2-YEAR-OLD DAUGHTER
THROUGH FERTILITY TREATMENTS)

What did our insurance cover? Zero. We felt very blessed that we were in the financial position to do go through treatments. It broke my heart every day when I was in the waiting room and I would be talking to all those women who would tell me things like they had to sell their house, and they had to do this and that and stop working and whatever it took. Some stopped working because they mentally couldn't do both [work and go through treatments]. Psychologically it was too much. The stories you hear in those waiting rooms are so heartbreaking. And I knew how blessed I was that at least I was able to financially do it the only way I was going to make it work.

CREBECCA, 50 (TTC FOR 4 YEARS; 4-YEAR-OLD BOY/GIRL
TWINS THROUGH FERTILITY TREATMENTS AND DONOR EGG)

Whether your insurance coverage is stellar or stinks, the finances related to treatment can add to the stress of infertility. Many insurance policies offer only limited options for

141

MONEY MATTERS

treatments, forcing dedicated baby-seekers to tap into their own savings. Although the American Society for Reproductive Medicine (ASRM) and the American College of Obstetricians and Gynecologists (ACOG) recognize infertility as a disease, the majority of states do not. As a result, most do not mandate that treatments be covered by insurance. It's considered an "elective" service (as if anyone in her right mind would ever "elect" to be infertile!). (See the Appendix for ways to become an agent to change these laws.)

If you pursued infertility treatments and were able to have at least some of the costs picked up by insurance, consider yourself lucky. Being covered isn't common (see "Who's Got You Covered?" on p. 140). This fact is blamed for keeping half of those who are experiencing infertility from pursuing treatment at all, especially more advanced techniques like IVF. Sadly, the high cost is a definite barrier for most couples.

Even if your insurance is decent, it likely doesn't cover every procedure, test, and medication for every single cycle. "Out-of-pocket" probably became a familiar refrain during your visits to the clinic, which left you with empty pockets a time or two. Even bills you thought would be covered by insurance might resurface months later, and you may find yourself battling with a claims adjuster—even after you have your baby. To set things straight, you may be stuck photocopying old bills, faxing off insurance cards, or navigating the maze of the insurance company's phone line and being placed on hold for hours—all of which takes time away from being with your baby.

playing to win

We live in Illinois, where there's mandated coverage for infertility treatment, and we had pretty good insurance. Even so, I'd say we spent about $120,000 total over *four years of aggressive treatment (including a couple of surgeries to remove fibroids, IUI rounds, and IVF), about $20,000 of which came out of our own pockets. That's a lot of money, but I was grateful we could afford it. It was worth it to me to work extra (I'm self-employed) to pay the medical bills. Our insurance covered four completed rounds of IVF and we did five total. I got pregnant several times but always miscarried. At that point, I was ready to quit treatment and adopt, and the fact that we'd exhausted our insurance coverage confirmed our decision.*

⌐KELLY, 41 (TTC FOR 6 YEARS; 2-YEAR-OLD SON
THROUGH DOMESTIC ADOPTION)

We probably spent close to $5,000 to $6,000 all together in this past year. We used the cash we had, because I'm pretty frugal.

I just realized I was throwing money at that fertility clinic. Three hundred dollars? No problem . . . then $500, $600. It just all became no big deal anymore.

⌐ASHLEY, 34 (TTC FOR 2 YEARS; PREGNANT WITH FIRST CHILD)

"Just give me one more chance!"

"I have a good feeling this time!"

"I'm due to win!"

Where are we in this scenario? In a Las Vegas casino or down at the fertility doctor's office, deciding whether or not to do another cycle?

For those who never established a date to end treatments, infertility can lead to behaviors similar to those with gambling problems. If you were obsessed with achieving pregnancy and found yourself in pursuit of your sixth IVF, your finances might not have had a chance to catch up, even after you give birth to or adopt your child.

You may have been swept up in the promises and the potential payoffs, and no naysayer could interfere with a silly thing like reason. (After all, there's nothing reasonable when it comes to infertility.) Did you begin hiding cycles from your extended family, hoping they wouldn't know that you were torturing yourself (not to mention your bank account) again by taking another risk? Maybe you borrowed from your retirement account, or hocked an heirloom. You were so preoccupied with the mission of a positive pregnancy test or sustaining a pregnancy, that you lost sight of the damage you were inflicting on everything around you, including your finances.

If you never gave a second thought to taking that second (or seventh) chance at IVF, you may find that in addi-

---

WHO'S PROFITING FROM INFERTILITY?

Want to get yourself really riled up about the economics of infertility? Check out *The Baby Business: How Money, Science, and Politics Drive the Commerce of Conception* by Debora L. Spar (Harvard Business School Press, 2006). She explores the topic of how fertility specialists are becoming increasingly creative in their financing plans, turning to loan programs, discount packages, shared-risk plans, and money-back guarantees to attract patients who without such options couldn't afford treatment. Selling the promise of parenthood is serving to enrich the clinics even further.

This book explores who's gaining financially from infertility (the clinics), who's suffering financially (wannabe parents) and what to do (institute more government regulation).

THE BELATED BABY

EGGS ON ICE

You have five choices when you go through infertility and have leftover embryos:

1. Use them (you can go through all of the motions as you did before; or you could ask your doctor for a "compassionate cycle" at little or no cost, where the embryos are put back into an unprepared uterus—just to bring yourself some closure).
2. Donate them for research (some programs will offer reimbursement of preservation costs if you do so).
3. Donate them to another infertile person.
4. Freeze them indefinitely. (This will cost you $500 per year. *Note:* A San Francisco woman gave birth to an embryo that had been frozen for thirteen years!)
5. Thaw them (a euphemism for "dispose of them").

tion to a baby, you also have a souvenir of debt from your infertility experience.

True—it's worth all of the money in the world to have your baby. But it's one thing to say that, and another to live with the fact that now it's time to pay up.

⌒ADOPTING ADDS UP

Coming up with $30,000 to begin with is challenging for most families. We'd really like to adopt. We just can't afford it.

⌒DAVINA, 36 (TTC FOR 8 YEARS; 1-YEAR-OLD DAUGHTER
THROUGH FERTILITY TREATMENTS)

To an infertility outsider, adoption is an obvious solution to your dilemma of how to build your family. There's no need to live a life without kids: "Just adopt!"

145

EMBRYO ADOPTION STARTING POINTS

If you can't bear the thought of discarding unused embryos but aren't actively seeking to become pregnant, check out the embryo adoption option. You may even receive reimbursement for previous storage fees if you donate.

- www.embryodonation.org
- www.miracleswaiting.org
- www.nightlight.org/snowflakeadoption.htm

But even if you're pro-adoption, you know that the financial barriers are significant—and are too great for every family to take on. The average adoption costs between $20,000 and $25,000, and coming up with that kind of cash can be a tremendous hurdle.

The costs associated with domestic adoption vary wildly. While adopting a child out of the foster care system is next to nil (averaging nothing to $2,500), this may not have been your first choice. The costs escalate from there. Adopting domestically can range from $5,000 to $40,000 and may include birth mother living expenses, depending on state law. Agency adoptions tend to be a little less expensive than private adoptions, but in either situation, there's always the chance that a birth mother will decide to parent—what caseworkers call "failed placements." You have no control over that happening, and the fact is that you may pay a well-intended birth mom thousands of dollars only to have her change her mind. You're out the money, with no baby to show for it.

You might be able to forecast more reliably how much an international adoption will cost, but even then there are unanticipated incidentals and fluctuations. You need to travel to a foreign country, sometimes more than once. The airfare, hotel, meals, cabs, and car rental fees add up quickly. On top of that, you may find yourself being coerced into paying the orphanage workers a "gift," in the form of cash or goods to stay in their good graces. Your excitement of adding to your family might feel tainted by feeling swindled at every turn.

In the end, though, you made it work and figured out a way to beg, borrow, or steal for the opportunity to adopt. Maybe you were creative and held a fundraiser. Maybe you slapped the entire bill on a zero-interest credit card and worked like a dog to pay it off before it came due. However you worked it out, you did, and you'd probably have paid double the amount for your child, knowing what you know now.

double whammy: infertility + adoption!

My husband was out of a job for a year, so we had to deplete a lot of our savings and then the fertility stuff further depleted some savings. We haven't had a chance to build that back up yet. And then before I got pregnant we started the adoption process and have spent like $6,000 to $7,000 dollars on that already. I mean, we're just cash-poor.

∾Lisa, 36 (TTC for 2 years; pregnant with first child)

According to RESOLVE, 65 percent of women who pursue infertility treatments wind up giving birth. To these people, the time and money spent on treatment was a solid investment.

But what happens to the other 35 percent whose investment doesn't pay off? They either choose a child-free existence, or pursue adoption.

If you chose the adoption route right away, you saved

ANY KID'LL COST YA

Forget about the high cost of getting pregnant or adopting a baby—there are all of the high costs associated with just being a parent! Depending on a family's income, raising a child can average between $134,000 and $285,000. From hospital bills through graduation ceremonies, it's clear that having kids is an emotional decision, not an economical one.

yourself some heartache—and some cash. But if you failed with treatments and then moved to adoption, you're in a double hole to start your parenting venture. This can be a frustrating financial situation, one that will influence your short-term and long-term future. For example, if the bills are overwhelming, you may be forced into returning to work when all you want to do is be home with your child. You may find that infertility is continuing to impact your life, even after the baby arrives.

⌒Double Jeopardy (or Triple, or Quadruple, or . . .)

When I told my boss that I was pregnant with triplets, she said, "Well, I'll start finding your replacement. I'm sure that you won't be coming back to work!" Infertility made the decision for me to become a stay-at-home mom—I didn't. When you consider the costs for a nanny or daycare for triplets, it just didn't make sense for both my husband and me to keep working. But then I started worrying about how much of a financial strain it was going to be with diapers, strollers, car seats, cribs, and college. The price of one kid alone is signifi-

cant—and then we had to multiply that by three, while dividing our income in half. It didn't compute!

⌐JILL, 38 (TTC FOR 3 YEARS; 7-YEAR-OLD GIRL/BOY/BOY
TRIPLETS THROUGH FERTILITY TREATMENTS)

When you find out you're pregnant with multiples after enduring infertility, it seems as though you've hit the jackpot. It's everything you've ever dreamed of—times two (or three, or more). But as the initial shock of the news wears off, you realize that your new "jackpot" is also going to deplete your pot of money.

Since multiple pregnancies are at a higher risk for having an unhealthy outcome, you may have to stop working sooner rather than later. This is especially true for those people who work non-desk jobs (i.e., nurses, flight attendants, waitresses, salespeople, etc.) and are on their feet frequently. When your doctor tells you to slow down and stay home, this may be hard if you're paid by the hour. Time off means money not earned. Bedrest costs.

If you're pregnant with multiples, you're also at a higher risk for complications that usually plague these pregnancies, such as pre-term labor, placenta previa, and pre-eclampsia. Unfortunately, no matter what great shape you're in, you're not exempt from developing problems. (Just as you weren't exempt from infertility!)

When you're pregnant with multiples, it's a fact that you're more likely to give birth early. How many weeks a baby is born prematurely is directly related to his odds of surviving and thriving. For example, a baby born at thirty-two weeks has a much better outlook healthwise than one born at twenty-five weeks. The earlier a baby is born, the more likely he is to stay in the hospital for an extended stay. As he develops his lungs and learns how to eat, those neonatal intensive care unit (NICU) line item costs can rack up in the hundreds of thousands of dollars you owe (if you lack coverage).

Even after your family is discharged from the hospital, the expenses keep multiplying. Depending on the health of your children, you might need to purchase or rent special equipment, like an apnea monitor or oxygen tank. You must succumb to buying a bigger vehicle to transport your brood around town, whether a gas-guzzling SUV or the dreaded and uncool (but less expensive) minivan. A brigade of strollers also fills your garage to the brim.

Speaking of garages, you might find that your house can't comfortably accommodate your new family, since it's more than doubled in size. When you're all of a sudden surrounded by swings, cribs, highchairs, and toys, the walls start closing in. You need more space. The bigger home you may have been considering buying five years from now suddenly becomes an urgent need.

When you have more than one baby, it seems as if people will come out of the woodwork to send gifts. At least when the babies are newborns, many people will show an outpouring of generosity. You're a novelty, and they want to be part of the baby action. Accepting certain handouts, however, might make you feel like you're the McCaughey septuplet family, who received a handout house, van, food, clothing, and diapers. While the public "oohed" and "ahhed" over the "miracle" of these seven babies, you might feel as if the septuplets are a spectacle to be pitied. Where's their pride for being self-sufficient?

Although you might welcome some financial relief, you might find accepting it is a double-edged sword. You do what's right for your family, but always in the back of your mind you know that it was infertility that strapped you with so many kids.

THE BELATED BABY

Infertility might continue to chip away at your pride (or maybe you have none left!).

⌒Hi Ho, Hi Ho, It's Off to Work You Go (. . . or No)?

As those years went by that I was infertile, I just felt more and more and more like I wanted to be a mom, that was just what I wanted to be. I had my career, I was happy with my career. But . . . I don't know. Maybe the infertility did crystallize that more, you know, make that feeling of wanting to be a full-time mom even stronger.

⌒Marisa, 37 (TTC for 4 years; 2-year-old boy/girl biological twins through fertility treatments)

It's the dilemma that every family faces—even our friends who are "fabulously fertile": Should both parents work, or should one of you forfeit the salary to stay at home with the kids? There are pros and cons to each scenario, and often, it's not an all-or-nothing decision. Many companies offer employees a flexible work schedule or part-time options these days, which eases the pain of being gone all day. There are also more opportunities to work from home than ever before, and if you can become a freelance something-or-other or sell enough Tupperware to your friends, you might be able to make ends meet.

Despite all of the alternatives that exist to full-time work, though, there's no denying that the highest paying jobs are full-time ones. Health insurance, retirement plans, and other perks of being part of a full-time roster might be things you just can't give up. The reality is that many families have no choice but to suit up and head out.

While there's no one right answer for every family's situation, you may not even realize how much infertility might influence which road you'll choose. And in some cases, infertility might just choose the road for you.

back to the briefcase

> *After going through infertility it's something I question—why I'm working full time. We had such a hard time having our daughter, why am I leaving her?*
>
> ⌐Kathleen, 42 (TTC for 3 years; 1-year-old daughter through fertility treatments)

> *I plan to go back to work, which kind of makes me feel bad. As much work as I've put into [having a child], I feel bad about going back to work instead of spending time with the baby. I plan on staying out twelve weeks, even though we really can't afford it.*
>
> ⌐Lisa, 36 (TTC for 2 years; pregnant with first child)

The party's over. The drama of infertility is behind you, and you're finally a complete family. Maybe there was no question all along that you would return to work after you brought your baby home.

There are plenty of reasons for returning to work, the most obvious one being that more income pays the bills! If it's too much financial pressure to rely on one paycheck, especially if you have leftover infertility debt, then it's natural for both of you to continue with your jobs. If you live in an area with a high cost of living (and you want to keep your home and feed your new kid), you may have no choice but to head back to the work world. With two incomes, there's also less pressure on either one of you to be the sole provider.

The benefits to both of you working aren't just financial either. You may find that, mentally, you aren't cut out for the full-time parent role. Your PhD means Ph-ooey to a pouting toddler, and you might miss the challenge that only full-time work offers. Not only are you avoiding feeling frustrated at home, but you are also fulfilling your own dreams—and serving as a role model to your child.

152

STAY-AT-HOME PAY?

Research by Salary.com shows that a stay-at-home mom's work is worth a whopping $138,095 per year. Considering her jobs as a housekeeper, cook, psychologist, day care center teacher, laundress, van driver, facilities manager, janitor, computer operator and CEO, this is what her total take-home pay would be.

Another study from Salary.com calculates that a stay-at-home dad's salaray would be $128,755. Why the discrepancy? Moms still put in longer hours, an average of 91.8 versus 80.2 for dads.

Ah, if only there was a place where you could collect that check!

Keeping your career in circulation also means you won't forfeit a future salary. For example, if you drop out of work now and decide to go back when your child is older, your salary might drop *as much as 37 percent* from what it would have been had you continued to work. Talk about a penalty!

vote for home

I appreciate [motherhood] more because I worked at it. I don't take it for granted so much. I'm not going back to work. I make almost twice as much as [my husband], and we're willing to cut down on that huge salary and make it on his salary just so I can be home, because we worked so hard at this. And I need to be with my baby.

—STEPHANIE, 40 (TTC FOR 7 YEARS; NEWBORN SON THROUGH FERTILITY TREATMENTS AND GESTATIONAL SURROGATE)

There's no denying that working outside the home pays. But there's also no substitute for being able to stay at home with your child if you're able to do so, financially and mentally.

Maybe you've waited for the opportunity to become a stay-at-home parent your whole life, and relish the opportunity to put your career aside for your kids. If you're older, you may have reached a point in your life where you've achieved success and now no longer feel the need to prove

FAMILY BUDGET BASICS

Don't break the bank when your kids come along! Gone are the days of DINK (double income, no kids). If you're now striving to live off of one income, note that a frugal family:

- eats in most nights, since frequently eating out or even ordering in adds up.
- buys in bulk and stashes extras in a freezer.
- breastfeeds, if possible, to save on formula costs.
- clips coupons, and then uses (versus loses!) them.
- finds toys and any "necessary" massive plastic items at garage sales.
- knows that generic labels (i.e., over-the-counter medicine, diapers, wipes) won't kill anyone.
- becomes a do-it-yourselfer whenever possible, making their own baby food, clothes, or curtains.
- cuts back on bells and whistles like souped-up cable channels or extra-speedy internet access.
- accepts and wears secondhand clothes.
- sells unused or lightly used items at their own garage sale or on eBay.

yourself. You are at peace with leaving your job, and want to focus all of your efforts on your kids. You're elated that you now have a reason to kiss the world of work goodbye and retire for good!

On the other hand, if you've always been a career-oriented person and never dreamed of quitting full-time work after kids, you may be surprised when infertility causes your outlook to shift. Through the years of not being able to be a parent, you might have gradually come to the realization that there's no more rewarding job in the world than being a parent, and it suddenly has become your sole priority. You feel the need to be there for your child full-time, all the time.

If you didn't experience such an epiphany, though, you may be feeling extreme guilt and forced into staying home. By working so hard at becoming a parent, you've been led to believe that you need to sacrifice the rest of your life because this is what you wanted so desperately. If you had multiples, you may feel as if you have no choice but to stay home. And if you adopted, you may feel pressure, whether it was unspoken or not, to become a stay-at-home parent. For example, if you told the birth parents that you were dying to be a stay-at-home parent, you may feel obligated to do just that, even if you're bored out of your mind doing so.

> *I looked on child rearing not only as a work of love and duty but as a profession that was fully as interesting and challenging as any honorable profession in the world and one that demanded the best that I could bring to it.*
>
> ⌒Rose Kennedy (1890–1995)

judgment from others

> *Many of [my infertility friends] have had the discussion about being a stay-at-home mom versus a working*

MONEY MATTERS

mom and, you know, most of us, especially living in a big city, a lot of us don't have much of a choice. We still have to work for finances. But just the emotional struggle that we face that some of us want to go back to work, which then has some conflict, because then there are some who say, "You've spent all these years in infertility, and now you're just going to go back to work?" Some of us want to go back to work. A lot of debates have taken place.

⌒DAVINA, 36 (TTC FOR 8 YEARS; 1-YEAR-OLD DAUGHTER
THROUGH FERTILITY TREATMENTS)

To work or not to work: This is the question everyone needs to decide, based on what's best for their own family.

So why do others feel the need to judge what we've decided? In some circles, there's an unspoken war that's being fought. It seeks to answer the unanswerable question: Who's the better parent, the one who stays home with the kids, or the one who works and therefore provides her family with more financial resources?

It's not fair, but infertility provides another avenue for others to judge what you decide. You are subjected to a double standard. After you sacrificed so much time, money, and emotional energy to build your family, how can you just up and go back to work? As an infertility survivor you may find that you're judged more harshly or to a higher standard than regular parents. You may feel even more selfish than "regular" parents if you decide to go back to work.

The key is to hash out the details with your partner and decide what's best for your family. No one else can decide what's right for you. Then, have confidence that you've made the right decision, and remember that you can always change your mind at a later point!

Now that you've succeeded at becoming a parent, your new role is to make sure that you plan your family's financial future adequately. Whether or not you've solved the "to work or not to work" dilemma, you need to dust off your documents and prepare to be a fiscally responsible parent.

Once you become a parent, you'll find that your previous budget has been blown to bits. From diapers and educational baby toys to summer camps and piano lessons, it's a given: this kid will set you back a few. (That's one thing you can definitely count on!)

baby basics

Right away, you'll want to apply for a social security number for your baby. No, you're not shipping him off to work quite yet. You're establishing your future entitlement to various tax credits you may be eligible to receive, such as child-tax credits and day-care credits, depending on your income. You may also want to review your paycheck and consider adding more allowances on your W4 form, to increase your take-home pay. While you're at it, make sure that your child is added to your health insurance and investigate purchasing additional life insurance offered through your employer, too.

where there's a will

Determining who will care for your children if you're unable to do so is one of the hangnails of a parent's financial tasks. Putting off creating a will is common—no one wants to think about kicking the bucket, after all—but the sooner you create this document, the sooner you'll have peace of mind.

Consider who might be best suited to care for your child if you're gone. Will she fare best with Aunt Susie, who has four kids of her own—or will bachelor Uncle Charlie in the city give her a better life and more attention? Much to the displeasure of their families, some parents select like-minded friends as a guardian option. Once you make your selection, be sure to ask the family if they're up for the job.

be smart: save for college

If you're struggling to figure out how you're going to pay your child's future college bill, you're not alone. The cost of a higher education has soared and keeps escalating. The College Board reports that the average tuition increase for 2007/2008 was 6.3 percent at private colleges and 6.6 percent at public universities over the previous year, outpacing both income increases and inflation rates. Despite this fact, *most parents have saved little to nothing* to cover future expenses, even though research shows they plan on paying some or all of the costs.

With so many variables, there's no one-size-fits-all when it comes to developing a savings strategy—except to start. Think of your savings program as a portfolio, which can be comprised of many investment components. In addition to an individual certificate of deposit or mutual fund account, add Roth IRAs, 529 plans (which you can purchase from any state) and state tuition plans into the mix to help save on federal and state taxes.

Also, remember to save enough. Putting away $25 a month might seem adequate when your child's a newborn, but you might need to bite a bigger bullet to make the grade. Depending on where your child will go to college (and if it's public or private), $300 a month might be more on target.

EDUCATE YOURSELF ON SAVINGS

- www.savingforcollege.com
- www.fastweb.com
- www.fafsa.ed.gov
- www.finaid.org
- www.acenet.edu
- www.collegesavings.org
- www.independent529plan.org

SPEND TO SAVE

Enrolling in credit card programs that put dollars away for school can be a sneaky way to add dollars to your child's college savings plan.

- www.futuretrust.com
- www.upromise.com
- www.babymint.com
- www.littlegrad.com

retirement

While it might be tempting to pull or borrow funds from your Individual Retirement Account (IRA), 401(k), or other qualified retirement plan to help cover some temporary kid costs, this could be a costly mistake. The penalties for early withdrawals from retirement programs can set you back at least 10 percent—and sometimes even more, depending on the reason for withdrawal, your tax situation, and your age. Not only is there a short-term loss, but you'll also forfeit any long-term interest you might have gained.

A financial planner can set you straight as to better financing options. This is especially important if you're an older parent, facing retirement and your child's college bills simultaneously!

159

⟳TRUE SACRIFICE

The first three IVFs that we did we paid for out of pocket [for the first child], so we didn't incur any debt, and then we did the same for the fourth IVF [for the second child]. After I got pregnant with my second child, people asked, "Oh, are you going to get a minivan now?" And it's like, "Well, no, we don't have any money left!" We spent it on trying to conceive. We've made sacrifices. I drive a ten-year-old car, we live in a smaller house on a busy street. We don't have a ton of luxuries. I mean, we're not poor, but we're not rich; we just did without some of those things that maybe we would've spent money on if we hadn't spent it on IVF.

⟳JoANNE, 37 (TTC FOR 4 YEARS; 3-YEAR-OLD DAUGHTER AND
5-MONTH-OLD SON THROUGH FERTILITY TREATMENTS)

[My wife] and I talked about finances when we were considering adoption. One thing that I can't even imagine people considering, just because I know how frustrating it is when you're trying to have kids, is to go into debt to have children. I would think that that would bring so much more strain and stress on the marriage and how that just would not be a favorable situation. I like to pay things off and have no debt whatsoever.

Last year, we spent around $24,000 out of pocket for fertility treatments. Sure, that's money we could have used for other things like adding to a college fund—you name it. But then again I look at these two precious little boys and I go, "Wow, I would have doubled that." I mean, it's just money, you know?

⟳GREG, 36 (TTC FOR 6 YEARS; BIOLOGICAL
1-YEAR-OLD TWIN SONS)

160

THE BELATED BABY

Most people understand what true sacrifice means only after their child is born—and let's face it, some people never understand! Since you've been through infertility, though, you are familiar with what it's like to live without both material and emotional luxury long before you ever met your child.

As a result of past, present, or future sacrifices that were thrust upon you by infertility, there have been positive rewards. You're more focused on what's really important in life—your child—not the cars, vacations, big homes, and other perks that could've been. You're able to sift through and recognize what's merely the small stuff and focus on the blessing of your new life as a parent. Think of what a positive example you're serving to your children by being a disciplined manager of your finances.

8

Your Family's Story:
TO TELL OR NOT—AND HOW?

We are at this kiddie pool and I am in the water near both my sons, David [then 6] and Philip [then 2]. This little boy points to Philip asks, "Is this your son?"

"This is my son and this is my son," pointing to David and Philip both.

"Why is his skin brown and his skin lighter?" he continues.

So I say, "David has a tan."

Then David kind of leans toward him with a fatherly tone and explains why he looks different: "I came from an orphanage and my brother came from my Mommy's tummy."

It was so cute, but it also kind of made me sad to hear him describe his beginnings as being from an orphanage. But I was glad to see him step up and answer the question so deftly himself.

—JULIE, 49 (TTC FOR 3 YEARS; 7-YEAR-OLD SON THROUGH INTERNATIONAL ADOPTION AND 3-YEAR-OLD "SURPRISE" SON)

When you become a parent, you become proficient in telling tales. With your bookshelf brimming with all of the childhood classics, Peter Rabbit, Mother Goose, and Dr.

163

Seuss stand at the ready to help you read early and often to your child.

You may also enjoy telling the occasional impromptu story to your child at night. As you weave real facts with fiction off the top of your head, however, you begin to understand the power of your position in telling your child about her origins. It's up to you to decide when to reveal how your family was created . . . or if you'll reveal it at all. Will you twist the truth or delay revealing it—at least temporarily, you tell yourself—for your child's sake? What about for your sake?

You know the bare, nonfiction version of how you came into each others' lives. Your child does not. She doesn't know how you debated whether or not to continue treatments—or that she lost a sibling due to your agonizing decision to selectively reduce. The two adoptions that fell through before hers was a success don't cause her to wake up at night and think, "what if?" And until you explain that she was created thanks in part (so to speak) to a donated egg or sperm, or both, she's blissfully unaware of her biological status.

If your child is young, the reality is that she's probably more concerned about what you're serving for dessert tonight than how she came to exist in the world. But you know that you need to prepare for the conversation about your fertility frustrations—and the full story of her birth—eventually. Whether she was adopted after being abandoned on a church's doorstep or created on your seventh and final IVF with donated sperm, she deserves to know the truth—if not now, eventually.

You're in charge of what she knows, when she'll know it—and how she'll find out. She also needs your help in figuring out how to present herself to the world, and to feel

164

proud of who she is and how she came to exist. All parents must help their children develop a strong sense of identity, but as an infertility survivor you might have additional challenges as well.

ᴄ Accept the Truth Yourself

You spent longer than you wanted to, or expected to, to become a parent. In fact, you may have been obsessed with it. After planning your next treatment cycle or home study for what seemed like forever, you then spent months—or years—waiting anxiously for your new arrival. Being obligated by so many activities and appointments kept you pretty distracted, and may have overshadowed some bigger issues lurking for you on the horizon.

> *The truth will set you free, but first it will make you miserable.*
>
> ᴄ James A. Garfield,
> twentieth U.S. president

Desperate for a baby, you redefined the meaning of "great lengths." In hindsight you realize that you turned to certain treatments that previously you thought you'd avoid like the plague (like maybe all of them!). Whether for personal, moral, or religious reasons, you never believed that you'd need to—or ever would—resort to advanced fertility medicines or international adoption. But, lo and behold, you may have.

The good news is that the creative treatment or adoption worked—you're a parent! The bad news is that you may not have had a chance to really come to terms with how you accomplished your goal, and as a result are struggling with how to share the information of how it all happened with your child. You were desperate then—and may be in denial now.

If you're biologically related to your child and your partner isn't, you'll need to be especially sensitive to his or

165

her personal timeline of acceptance. It's easy to deal with donated eggs or sperm in the abstract. When it transforms into live flesh, bones, and personality, new feelings may evolve—even ones you thought you had dealt with already.

Don't be surprised when consequences of your infertility arise and rear their ugly heads. A small part of you might still long to be one of those "regular" parents pushing a stroller around town, but accept the fact that you'll never be one. You're an infertility survivor—and everything you've experienced makes you a special kind of parent.

Mourn the fact that things weren't perfect, and then find the strength to rise above it. The situation isn't about you any longer. You've brought a person to life or into your life, and it's about her now. Recognize that one of your child's needs is for her to know the full history of how she came to be.

⌒The Simplicity of the Truth

I don't like hide things from any of my kids; I'm very open when appropriate. I don't believe in secrets in the closet. They know how they were conceived, they know Dr. Doyle, they know that they were in a test tube. I think I talked about it more when they were younger; now, I think sometimes . . . I think the boys know and sometimes they forget, but I kind of go over it and they'll say, "Mom, why are you telling me this?" I think it's important, though. And children are very, very perceptive.

⌒Karen, 47 (TTC for 6 years; 13-year-old daughter and 9-year-old twin sons through fertility treatments)

If you're a Dear Abby fan (or merely a reader—like a car crash, you can't look away from the column), at some point you've probably run across a letter from a teen who's

THE BELATED BABY

just found out for the first time that he's adopted. Keeping him in the dark for over a decade, his adoptive parents didn't have the heart—or the guts—to inform him of his background any sooner. Whether to protect him from feeling inferior due to his adoption or to shield him from possible rejection from his biological parents, the adoptive parents had performed a cover-up worthy of an international CIA operative. As a result, the teen rebels and goes out searching for his "real" parents. Of course, he fantasizes they will be more permissive and understanding of his problems than his current family could ever be.

Did those adoptive parents make a colossal mistake in keeping hush-hush, since the teen is in such turmoil? Possibly. You pledge not to fall into the same trap, hoping more than anything to cultivate an environment of openness in your family right from the start. Unlike adoptive parents in previous generations, you have every intention of sharing the full story of your child's birth with her. But when do you start?

the age of enlightenment

When is the "right" age to tell your child the truth about his birth? It would be nice if someone would invent a handy "psychologically approved timetable," magnetized for the fridge, to guide parents through this all-important task. Unfortunately, there's no magical age when it's the right time to share the details of your child's birth with him. Each family's truth is as unique as its members; there's no formula to apply to all situations.

One thing that *is* a common denominator in all situations is a child's age and ability to comprehend an explanation. A two-year-old isn't able to grasp the technical details of her birth; a happy, high-level mention of infertility or adoption may be all that's needed at this age. As your child

BABY STEPS TO YOUR STORY

Do you love kissing, holding, and singing to your infant, but feel ridiculous "just talking" to her? Don't! Babies love hearing the sound of their parents' voices. As you merrily tell your baby about her surroundings and what day of the week it is, consider covering the topic of her creation while it's still fresh in your mind. Telling your infant that she is "part dad, part helpful lady with the good eggs" might sound over-the-top, but with practice you'll find the words that perfect your message—and also make it positive. Sharing the information doesn't take anything away from you as her parent, but instead puts you in the position of sharing the beauty of how your child was created with her.

grows, however, so will the questions and complexities. A five-year-old might be fascinated with the story and ask more questions than you'd care to answer. As long as you keep the conversation from becoming too technical or in any way negative, you're on the right track.

You'll probably find that as you steadily repeat your message *throughout* the years, more and more age-appropriate details will surface. While you might feel uncomfortable divulging how IVF is different from having babies the "regular" way to your four-year-old, for example, your teen is more than ready to engage in this conversation. (Well, maybe *you* still won't be ready, but nevertheless, it's the right time!)

right from the start
Just as a "regular" parent talks to her kid about how she craved pickles during pregnancy, non-biological parents

have just as many (or more!) stories up their sleeves to share. Let's face it: Any story that you tell your child that involves him and how he came to be will be fascinating to him. Maybe the birth mother went into labor in the middle of the night and you drove seven hours straight to the hospital and almost ran out of gas—making it just in time as he was making his grand entrance into the world.

In telling (and endlessly retelling) his unique story to your child, the truth simply becomes part of your family's lore. There'll be no need for a dramatic huddle to reveal the

---

PASSING ON THE PAIN?

If our child's right to information about his biological parents is denied, are we simply passing on the pain of our own infertility woes to him?

While there are laws to protect the rights of children worldwide, including ones that protect their rights to their identity, many anonymous donation practices seem to run counter to those ideals.

---

big news after your seven-year-old blows out the candles on his birthday cake. If you incorporate the stories of how your family was created into your daily life and throughout the years, your child will understand and be proud of his background—and be well-adjusted and happy.

When the truth is accepted and integrated into your family's life all along, you'll most likely find that it's a non-event that doesn't really impact you on a daily basis. There are bills to pay and soccer games to play, after all. You're not sitting around rehashing and relishing in all of the fertility disclosure around you!

169

Even if you've been forthright from the get-go, don't be modest about your honesty. Be proud of yourself for your truthfulness. There's a sense of freedom for families who have no skeletons. There's space to grow in a room that's not full of elephants.

⌒Spectrum of Secrecy

My husband wanted to keep the fact that we were using a donor egg very quiet. He felt like it was completely nobody's business. I felt, on the other hand, that I had to share it with my girlfriends. If you have a secret, it festers. It becomes bigger. Scarier. Nastier.

We're not sure how we're going to tell our daughter. It's been a very polarizing topic of conversation between me and my husband. I know she needs to know who her birth mother is if health issues come up . . . but she does look just like her dad. Right now we're taking what I call a "vague" approach. She's only two. We don't talk

---

TO TELL OR NOT TO TELL

In Sweden, all children conceived through donor insemination have a right to know the identity of the donor. A study of parents there with children created via donor insemination found that 61 percent of them had told their child the news when they were around five years old. The others? They were afraid of other people's attitudes, and felt that it was private information. (They were also less educated than couples choosing identifiable donors.) So while it's the law to tell, ensuring compliance seems to be another challenge.

THE BELATED BABY

about it, I guess. I don't know how we're going to tell her
. . . or if we will.

⌐Claire, 42 (TTC for 3 years; 3-year-old daughter
through fertility treatments and donor egg)

Of course, some truths are easier to tell than others.

When you're parenting a child who's a different race from your own, the fact that you adopted her might be obvious. You might not like it one bit when strangers come up to you and ask you where you adopted your daughter from, but this doesn't break the news to your daughter that she's Chinese. Likewise, if you're in a same-sex partnership, the biological facts of your family are "out"; it's no mystery that there was some creativity involved with her conception! Your child lives with the fact, or at least with a few clues, that she is somehow different.

But what if your infertility "truth" isn't hard to hide? Will you attempt to hide it?

If you're part of the 31 percent of adoptive parents who've never met the birth parents, you may be tempted to be tight-lipped about the past—or at least to try to gloss over it. Likewise, coming clean about using donor egg or sperm poses a challenging reproductive conundrum. (Just as many wonder if a tree falling in a forest makes a sound if no one's around to hear, does not discussing your child's biological background really make a difference?)

Maybe you always believed that you'd tell your child the full story of his birth, but you find that as the years go by, you don't. The topic never seems to come up; never mind that's because you never bring it up.

The belief that you're protecting your child from emotional pain is a major reason why you might be reluctant to let the facts fly. You might be afraid of being rejected by your child. Or maybe you're just plain busy. Like any other

171

parent, you're immersed in school, church, and sports activities, and you find that there's no convenient time to fit the "heavy duty discussion" into your schedule.

You know deep down, though, the ethical responsibility to tell your child the truth depends on you. It's a human, fundamental right for people to know their genetic background. It's critical not only from the standpoint of having access to their genetic history for health reasons, but for their emotional well-being as a person.

social acceptance

If thinking about sitting down with your child for a talk causes you to squirm, keep in mind that the social stigmas associated with adoption, surrogacy and donor births have come a long way since July 25, 1978, when the first "test-tube" baby Louise Brown was born in the United Kingdom. Short of cloning (although for $200,000 or more, you can wait in line for that, too), few reproductive feats shock peo-

172

ple these days. We've grown accustomed to hearing about reproductive marvels on a daily basis, from sextuplets being born to sixty-seven-year-old women giving birth to twins. Whether due to the advanced technologies or the increased volume, creatively conceived babies are more socially accepted than ever before.

Fortunately, these miracle births are celebrated as joyous occasions. For as judgmental as some people can be, there's something about a real, live, baby in the flesh that tends to unify others and melt even the hardest of hearts.

shame on your child? shame on you!

If you're having trouble mustering up enough confidence to break the news to your child that he's not biologically related to you, consider the worst-case scenario of failing at this task. At age seventeen, he'll find out from some random aunt or friend's parent that he was adopted, freak out, and run away from home in search of his birth parents. He'll vow never to speak with you again. You've shattered his self-confidence, caused him to doubt his identity, and made him feel ashamed of who he is—all by not telling him the truth.

Okay, that sounds more like the plot of a *Lifetime* movie. But doesn't this forecast sound a lot worse than you being slightly uncomfortable at the kitchen table for about, say, eleven minutes, when your child is four years old?

Think about how you would want to receive the news that you know you need to deliver. What do you want to hear? Maybe your message includes that your child was surrounded by so many loving people who wanted him to be born (you and your spouse, the doctor, and the donors), and everyone worked together as a team to make sure that happened. If you met one or both of the birth parents, tell him so, and say something positive about each one.

173

Once you get going and speak from your heart, you'll most likely find that the truth is pretty easy to tell. Most importantly, your child will know without a doubt that you're on his side and will always be a trusted person in his life.

You can be trusted for the truth.

positive reactions

We definitely have shared [the fact that our twins were conceived via donor egg] with our family and extended family, because we firmly believe there should not be family secrets. We knew that we would be telling our kids from day one. From the minute they were born, we told them about the special lady that helped us. They've heard about that their whole life. And they understand more and more over the years.

We did tell some close friends. Sometimes it gets a little awkward, because I'll forget which friends I've told and which friends I didn't. And one of them might make a comment, "Oh, [your son] does that just like you," or whatever, and I wonder, does she know, does she not know?

I feel like it's my kids' information. It should be up to them who they share it with. It's nobody's business. But I don't want them to feel ashamed of it, either.

⌒ANITA, 43 (TTC FOR 4 YEARS; 7-YEAR-OLD TWIN SONS THROUGH FERTILITY TREATMENTS AND DONOR EGG)

Kids have a way of picking up on our own insecurities. Don't fool yourself: Your child has some pretty keen senses and knows if you're feeling negative or apprehensive about anything. This means that if you enter into conversations about your child's background with a matter-of-fact, positive attitude, odds are in your favor that your child will respond cheerfully, too.

174

Watch that your words aren't too complex, and keep a relaxed smile on your face. Leave the anxiety you felt during infertility out of the conversation, and instead bring the exuberance and enthusiasm you felt when your child came into your life.

Not surprisingly, one study of four- to eight-year-olds who were told that they were the result of donor inseminations found that the kids were either very curious about this fact or completely disinterested! Based on your child's per-

LESSONS FROM ADOPTED ADULTS

What better resource to know what your child might be feeling than to talk with an adopted "kid" who's all grown up? For insight on what your child might be feeling about his adoption and guidance on how to prepare for questions and feelings, consider talking to a few adopted adults. Adoption isn't a recent arrangement. From Moses floating down the Nile River in the Bible to today, there are far more than a few adopted adults floating around in the world. About 60 percent of people have a personal connection with adoption; either knowing someone who was adopted, having adopted a child, or having relinquished a child for adoption.

Explain that you would value their input with helping your adopted child, and ask (or email!):

- What was the best thing about being adopted?
- What was the worst thing about being adopted?
- Would you have changed how you received the news that you were adopted?
- What was the best thing your parents told you about your adoption? Was there a special story that they told?
- Is there anything that you wish could've been different?

PAGING DONOR #444

When you adopt or use donor eggs or sperm, your child's birth story will forever involve someone else. Even if you and the donors thought you had made up your minds to keep the adoption closed or the donation anonymous, your child (or donor) might have other plans in the future.

For the first time in history, birth parents, donors, and offspring who were in a closed situation can start sleuthing in order to piece together their own biological history.

With the Internet at everyone's fingertips and powerful, populated databases at the ready, people are finding new biological connections every day:

- www.donorsiblingregistry.com
- www.dcnetwork.org
- www.amfor.net
- www.adoption.com

This is a new frontier for our society, one that is continuing to evolve. Reconnecting offspring with donors—and even siblings of the same donor—is a reality. Denying the possibility won't change that!

sonality, it might be easy to predict which way he'll take the news.

Whether your child will be curious or couldn't care less, the important thing is to "just do it." No matter how old your child is today, it's never too early—or too late—to tell him the truth. Just plan what you need to say, find a good time to deliver the news matter-of-factly, and listen with your ears—and your heart—to your child's reaction and feelings.

I have recently been debating when to tell Philip that his brother, David, was adopted. I don't think he will really understand it, and my fear is that he will bring it up at an inopportune time and it could embarrass David. So far, David does not seem at all self-conscious about being adopted (he's usually quite matter-of-fact about it), but I think most kids want a bit more privacy about it as they get older, and they want to share that info themselves, as they see fit. So while we don't hide the fact of David's adoption and we speak freely about it, we haven't actually sat down to tell Philip. We will soon, I think.

◯JULIE, 49 (TTC FOR 3 YEARS; 7-YEAR-OLD SON THROUGH INTERNATIONAL ADOPTION AND 3-YEAR-OLD "SURPRISE" SON)

Even if you haven't told your child about his origins yet (but you're planning on it, right?), chances are that at least a few people already know about your fertility struggles and how your child came into your lives. Parents who have adopted or used donors almost always give family or friends at least a few clues as to what's going on.

If you're apprehensive about facing the truth head on, it's wise to let your inner circle of people in the know grow gradually, starting with your immediate family. Naturally, you'll want your child's siblings to understand how your family was created. It's part of their history and identity too, after all! However they themselves were created, creatively or biologically, tell them the same story you told their brother or sister. Be sure to use age-appropriate information, too. At the same time, tell the sibling his own birth story, too, so he doesn't feel left out.

As you feel more comfortable explaining your child's origins to him, you'll begin to trust more friends with the

177

information, too. Ask them to be sensitive with the information, and to use care when they share. While you don't need to keep your child's origins top secret, you also don't need to advertise it all over town, either!

Living in fear of who knows what about your kids and what will be divulged by the keg during the next block party is a tough way to live. If you manage the message carefully, you'll have no need to worry about any unplanned announcements. When you live openly and honestly, you're able to preserve the trust between you and your children.

⌒CRAFTING YOUR FAMILY'S "MESSAGE"

We have started saying, "We adopted him at birth" instead of "He's adopted." I heard another adoptive parent explaining how he and his wife use that language because it explains how their son joined their family instead of labeling him. (They have two children, one biological and one they adopted when he was ten days old.) Now I automatically say "we adopted him," instead of "he's adopted." It sounds like a minor thing, but it matters to me—and I want Ryan to grow up hearing that language, not feeling like "the adopted kid."

⌒KELLY, 41 (TTC FOR 6 YEARS, 2-YEAR-OLD SON THROUGH
DOMESTIC ADOPTION)

Even though you and your family don't need to run out and hire a public relations firm, it's a good idea to give some thought as to what your family's story is ahead of time. This gives you time to hone and practice it, which will serve not only to reassure every family member, but also to give you all the confidence to face the world.

Once you start talking about the facts openly within

THE BELATED BABY

your immediate family, you'll find that the message begins to shape itself. The tricky part may come in putting a slight spin on the truth or delicately creating a "white lie" where needed. For example, if you know that your child's biological parents were troubled drug-addicted teens, it might take

INSTEAD OF SAYING . . .	TRY SAYING . . .
"Your real mother gave you up for adoption—she just couldn't afford you."	"Your birthmother loved you so much, she wanted you to grow up in the best home possible."
"When you were a baby, you lived in an orphanage."	"Caretakers who loved you and other babies lived together in a place called [Insert name of group home].
"We used IVF with a donated ovum and Daddy's sperm to create an embryo."	"To start growing you, we needed two cells. One came from Daddy and another came from a helper. Then the cells went into Mommy's tummy."
"We used fertility drugs, which caused hyperstimulation, too many follicles and a multiple birth."	"We used special medicines and were so happy when we got an extra helping of babies from God!"
"Your birth mother left you wrapped in a blanket in a laundry basket, left outside on someone's front stoop."	"Your birth mother probably watched the family's house for days and made sure you were in a safe place. I have a feeling that she knew right where we would find you."

extra effort on your part to view the situation with rose-colored glasses. While the payoff to you was that you received a beautiful baby, your baby needs to hear something reassuring about himself in the story. Did the teens love each other? Was one a football star or a cheerleader? These are the kinds of positive details that your child will cling to, and won't take anything away from his identity.

No matter how old your child is when you tell her about her birth, the most important thing to remember is to always be positive—and to be yourself. Your love and honesty will shine through, no matter how tough the talks turn.

ᗡJUST WHOSE BUSINESS IS IT, ANYWAY?

> *My mother-in-law works in a gift shop and I brought [my son] in a few weeks ago. This other woman said to me, "Oh, where did he get his big brown eyes from?" I kind of looked at her because I thought she knew he was adopted. And I said, "Well, he got them from his birth father."*
>
> *And she kind of just shut her mouth and walked to another part of the store. My mother-in-law said, "Oh my—[she] felt so bad!"*
>
> *I'm like, "Why? It's really not a big deal, I'm not trying to hide anything. And that's where he got his big brown eyes from!"*
>
> ᗡDENISE, 45 (TTC FOR 5 YEARS; 2-YEAR-OLD SON
> THROUGH DOMESTIC ADOPTION)

Your family's story will morph over time and eventually evolve into handy, portable quips. While you don't need to buy a megaphone and shout the story from the rooftops, you are safe in knowing that you are prepared for the questions that will come your way. You're now ready to deliver them to people who feel a need to be "in the know."

That's not to imply, however, that anyone who asks is

automatically entitled to your full family history. There's a wide range in truth, from the high-level (my son was adopted from Guatemala) to the nuttiest grain (we failed ten IVF cycles and it took three years to adopt). Remember: you should never feel obligated to share anything with anyone. It's a delicate balance of what you share, with whom, and when.

Above all else, you should avoid making your child feel any shame about his origins. Share and provide full disclosure in situations when it's appropriate, which will make your child feel comfortable, too. At the same time, even if you don't feel ashamed by your infertility and are happy to discuss the details with anyone who passes by, your child might not be at the right age to be that much in the know. Pick your moments carefully.

In order to shield your kid from all of the insensitive blobs out there (who, of course, somehow themselves managed to be born!), you might feel a strong urge to run off and hole up at an isolated ranch in Idaho. Since this is probably infeasible and not what you really want, you must face the fact that you share the world with others. And, without a doubt, these others have questions. Sometimes they are personal, sometimes they are sensitive and there are always way, way too many of them.

To leave peacefully, strive to answer people's questions with the same matter-of-fact attitude that you might with your child. In fact (and especially when your child is with you), it's a good idea to use the same story and phrases that you do when talking with your child about his beginnings. When you repeat the story verbatim, your message is reinforced and becomes ingrained in your family members' minds. Your child is also then slowly equipped with how to handle inquisitive strangers solo, if needed.

181

Always remember: Your child is watching your every move. Yes, that stranger's comments were rude. But even if you think your grimace or narrowing of your eyes weren't visible, you kid knows when you're perturbed. In fact, she probably knows better than anyone—especially more so than that rude stranger!

Although you might dread the questions that are com-

CLEVER COMEBACKS

Sometimes you're in the mood to share your family's history with strangers, and sometimes you just want to enjoy a restaurant in peace. But if you're one of those "obvious infertiles," people might perpetually badger you to explain how your family came to be.

If you act bothered or are rude, your child might start to associate how she was created as something negative. Instead, try using a cheerful disposition as you deliver clever comebacks, such as:

- Nosy question: "Are you the grandma?" (You're an older parent). Comeback: "Me? Oh no! [TRY TO LAUGH] I'm just a mom who's a little late out of the parenting starting gate, but I'm keeping up just fine!"
- Nosy question: "Were you on fertility drugs?" (You're surrounded by kids the same age in a restaurant). Comeback: "We needed some extra help conceiving—and now we could use some help taking care of our quads. Will you please pass the ketchup?"
- Nosy question: "Where did he come from?" (Your child looks different from you). Comeback: "Like all children, he's a gift from God—and his Guatemalan birth mother."

UNFUNNY JOKES

When people joke about their kids being adopted or siblings tease one another that one of them was adopted—we all have brown eyes but yours are blue, so you must be adopted—it may hurt your feelings. Unfortunately, you just need to develop a thicker skin. As a matter of fact, you may have joked like this before you became an infertility survivor yourself.

Be gentle with the insensitive types; although you didn't sign up for the job, you play an important role in educating them.

ing your way today and or will soon come your way in the future, it's an inevitable part of your lives. Use your encounters with strangers as an opportunity to set a positive, direct example when dealing with people, and before you know it, your kid will be following your lead.

9

Trying Again:
ADDING ANOTHER CHILD TO YOUR FAMILY

IF YOU TRIED long and hard to have a child, you probably made lots of prayers—and promises. "Just give me one healthy baby, and I'll be happy."

And you meant it. But guess what? Despite those promises and what you truly believed while in the throes of trying to have your first baby, there's a good chance that you'll want to add another little person to your family. According the U.S. Census Bureau's demographic data from 2000, the average family size is 3.14 (perhaps this holds some kind of clue into solving pi).

Yet you might find it daunting to even consider going through the process to hold baby number two—especially if you're still diapering baby number one. Those same old worries that you encountered during infertility will surface again: What's our strategy? How long do we try? How much do we spend? For those who adopt, the second-time-around process might also pose some extra hurdles or eliminate certain adoption options that were available previously.

While you'll encounter some of the same dilemmas that you did while in pursuit of your first child, there will be an added twist: You must consider your new family's needs above everything else now, and what's best not only for you and your spouse, but also for your child.

Even if you were blessed with multiples out of the infertility gate, how do you *really* know when your family is complete? (There are plenty of families out there with three, four, or more children, after all.) And with science pushing us to the brink of new possibilities—hey, these days sixty-six-year-old women can birth twins!—could the answer be, we never really know?

ᗒFAMILY FANTASY

I always wanted four children, but I didn't have the choice. I mean, I'm so thrilled that I have my beautiful family and here I am saying "Oh, I want more!" Can't I just be happy with what I have? I should be thankful that I have three kids. But you know, whenever there's a pregnant woman, or I see a new baby, I would love to have had the option to say, "Hey, I want to have a baby." That's not an option for me. And now that I'm in my wonderful late forties, it's definitely over and that's okay. But you know, [the feeling of wanting another child] can still sneak up on you.

ᗒKAREN, 47 (TTC FOR 6 YEARS; 13-YEAR-OLD DAUGHTER AND
9 YEAR-OLD TWIN SONS THROUGH FERTILITY TREATMENTS)

When we were kids, many of us had a magic number in mind as to how many kids we'd have when we grew up and had our own families. Maybe that number was eleven. Maybe it was two. Maybe it was zero. Often that number was similar to our family size growing up, and probably just as often it was the opposite of our experience growing up (i.e., if your family was small, dreams of an extra big one were appealing).

186

Thinking about the gender of those kids was fun, too. Remember playing the board game Life? There was something pretty darn neat about landing on the boy/girl twin square and putting a pink and blue plastic stick into the slots of the car game piece. It felt efficient and complete to have "one of each."

Before marriage and in the early stages of it, you probably talked with your partner about how many kids you'd have, how far apart they'd be born (and of course, how cute they all would be). Those baby fantasies were fun, but you took them seriously. And it was all figured out, until infertility struck.

Unlike the perky neighbor whose family building plans came to perfect fruition, your family hasn't been able to follow that original blueprint. Remembering your "original" family plans has become difficult, since the dream was

---

AN "ONLY" NOT SO LONELY

Today there are approximately 14 million "only children" in the United States, according to the U.S. Census Bureau. The percentage of only children compared to all kids has more than doubled in the past twenty years, up from 10 percent to over 23 percent. About one-third of all American families started today will have a one-child family. But this number doesn't reveal how many of those families have singletons by choice, and how many would have liked to have more kids but were unable to. (The average age when a woman has her first child is almost twenty-five, compared to twenty-one in 1970, shortening the window of childbearing years.)

blown to bits. And gender? Pink, blue—purple—you'd take anything!

Since infertility has already dissolved your previous dreams, you may have had to reinvent your idea of the ideal family and come up with a new idea of normal. Today, you might be wondering if one is "good enough" for you; after all, you have a beautiful—and hopefully healthy—child at last. But if this only whets your appetite for more children, you might be even more reluctant to let go of your dreams for more.

☙ONLY CHILD FACTOR

There are forty-five kids on my street, and there's only one other household that has one child. That's because the mother died. So, it's a single dad and his child. Everyone else has a brother or sister situation, and you know, we tried, and it didn't work.

Teachers assume there's a younger or older sibling at home. The kids are often assigned different projects where you have to bring in pictures of your family. My son feels left out and just plain different by this some-times.

☙MARGARET, 47 (TTC FOR 6 YEARS; 9-YEAR-OLD SON
THROUGH FERTILITY TREATMENTS)

The first chapter of the Bible instructs us to "be fruitful and multiply," and (Lord knows) we've done our best to do just that over the years. But after having "just" one, does that math count as multiplying? More importantly, can you be satisfied with "just" one child in your life?

There are loads of stereotypes about only children, many of which aren't nice. There's the belief that because they monopolize their parents' attention, they're spoiled brats who must be at the center of everyone else's attention.

Without siblings, the usual give-and-take process of how relationships work is absent, and they wind up unable to relate well with their peers. Also, people think that since these kids are around adults all of the time, they have a tendency to become too "adult-like." Then there's the spoiled factor—the only kid gets everything he or she wants only to grow up and become a self-indulgent, self-absorbed brat. Who wants to parent (or even be around) a person like this?

The truth is, though, that only children do just fine. In fact, they do better than fine, outscoring their peers with siblings, at least academically. Research by the Office of Educational Research and Improvement shows that, like first-borns, only children score higher on measures of intelligence and achievement. Socially, while only children are perceived to have difficulty with same-age playmates and to act too adult-like, their scores on popularity and self-esteem have the same mixed results as those of children who have brothers or sisters. The myths are busted.

Also, unlike kids who must compete for their parents' attention, only children can bask in the glow of theirs. Many families of only children report a strong bond between each other, and feel closer as a result of their smaller size. There's nowhere to hide from one another in a small family if you're feeling down.

In addition to the extra attention and dedication, only children are the benefactors of the finances of the family. While this is may not be a morally redeeming perk for most people, its benefit is undeniable. Vacations for three are more attainable than those for four or more, so an only child might have more opportunities to see the world than his friends who are saddled with siblings. College for one? Expensive, but not impossible. Of course, having one kid

189

costs more than no kids, but the bottom line is less than two or more.

In addition to the upside of extra attention and money, many parents of one take pride in the fact that they're part of the solution to save our planet from the negative results of overpopulation. The fewer people there are in the world, the better chance we all have at a higher quality of life. Talk about keeping an eye on the big picture!

But this presumes that you want to parent one child. If that's the case, you may not even be reading this chapter! If you want more children, though, or are still on the fence, you're probably anxious about how you'll complete your family—or how to decide on the "right" family size.

⌒THE CASE FOR MORE

I'm an only child and had to deal with my mom's situation all alone. She had Alzheimer's, was placed in a nursing home, and recently passed away. I was the one who had to make the funeral arrangements. Because of all of this, I'm particularly sensitive to not wanting [my son] to be an only child.

⌒DAWN, 36 (TTC FOR 3 YEARS; 3-YEAR-OLD BIOLOGICAL SON)

While there are pros to keeping your family small, there are other strong reasons for wanting to pursue more children. The ability to shower your child with one-on-one attention is wonderful, for example, until you're ready to cook dinner, pay bills, or just veg out. As your child grows, you might start to feel like Julie, the cruise director from the *The Love Boat,* in a constant state of planning activities and playdates. You might overcompensate for not wanting your child to ever feel lonely—although this is something that can happen even in a family of ten!

The constant attention might also lead you to worry

more, and pin all your hopes and dreams on your one child. Your quest for the perfect schedule, perfect academic record, and perfect parenting decisions might take over, and end up putting excessive pressure not only on your little person but on you, too.

Along the same lines, parents of one sometimes have more acute fears that something will happen to their only child. Every parent wants their child to be safe, but with an only child, the sense of danger is compounded by the "if anything happens, that's it" mentality. Each bump, tumble, or trip to the emergency room can become that much more of a crisis when your family is small.

Parents of one are more aware than most that each stage of childhood is precious, so it can become intensely poignant when each one passes. Once you're done with diapers, you're really done with diapers. While parents with multiple kids might cast off those rompers with the snap-crotch with a shrug, the parent of one is often more reluctant to let go. They know once the time is gone, it's gone forever. As a result, they might linger with each new transition and unwittingly baby their preschooler. Without a younger sibling coming up in the wings and taking over the baby role, it's hard for a parent to let go and move on.

Finally, there's the fear that as an adult, your child will be obligated to care for you—his older parents—without the support of a sibling. This worry is even more real if you were an older parent to begin with, due to infertility. You love taking care of your baby, but you don't want the day to come when your baby has to take care of you—and maybe your husband, too—all by herself. Isn't that too big of a burden?

No matter what the motivation, whether to provide your child with a sibling or spare him from a future of being alone, it's a personal decision of whether to add to your family. If it feels as though there's someone missing in your family, whether you have one child or four, those feelings of being incomplete are real.

ᴗWHEN YOU AND YOUR SPOUSE DON'T AGREE

We talked, argued, debated for a couple of hours that night. He told me that he wants to make his life simpler, not more complicated. I told him that if I had one dream for the next decade it would be to raise another child. He told me that he would rather leave the marriage than do that, and that if it really was such a big dream, he could move down the street and I could do it on my own.

Let's just clarify my dream here. Following my dream does not entail destroying my marriage, creating a broken family for my son, and becoming a single mom. No. My dream is to adopt as a family—mother, father, and brother.

But here's my problem, which I'm sure is self-evident: How do I deal with the emotions that are left behind? How do I reconcile that someone else is making the decision for me to give up my dream?

ᴗPATRICIA, 43 (TTC FOR 4 YEARS; 7-YEAR-OLD SON
THROUGH FERTILITY TREATMENTS)

There are strong reasons for having more children—and there are strong reasons for having an only child. So what happens when you and your spouse feel strongly, but in opposite directions?

You've already gone through infertility, which strains even the healthiest of marriages. Now you've got that precious baby and, guess what? It's stressful, too. Making the effort to get back to sleepless nights and stinky diapers may

192

seem counterintuitive to the more pragmatic partner, who's most concerned with keeping the family on a schedule and a budget. The second time around, you must also consider how your child will adapt and relate with the new child, especially if you're adopting an older child into your family. And then there's the expense of it all.

The fact is that there will always be reasons—compelling ones—not to have more children. But only you (and your partner) can weigh the reasons and make the decision that's right for your family.

In addition to all of the "normal" stressors that go into deciding whether or not to have another child, there's also the infertility stress if you are facing treatments again. (Maybe this is why one partner has changed his mind about your family's size. Have you talked about it?) You've both been through it before, and the thought of going through it all again might be overwhelming and depressing. You're more knowledgeable about the process—but that's not necessarily a good thing. Only the two of you can decide whether this knowledge gives you the power you need to pursue it all again.

Marriage is a constant compromise, but this issue is a biggie. It cuts deeper than most decisions since it has everlasting implications. To bridge the impasse, it might be helpful to seek the advice of a professional counselor. A counselor's outside point of view gives you the ability to conduct productive conversations together. Hashing out the hesitations and discussing the reasons behind wanting more children will lead to the right decision for your family.

So why go to the trouble? For all the same reasons you both went to the trouble to have your first child. Or you may decide to keep your family the size it is, and that's fine too. This is a personal decision, so if you've always wanted to have one child, don't let anyone make you feel guilty about your little "lonely only." Have an answer at the ready to ward off nosy questions about when you're going to have another one, and don't apologize. Hanging out with other parents with similar family structures can offer additional support (and moms who probably feel the way you do, too.)

⌁FEELING GREEDY

If you both decide to give this second (or third, or fourth) child a chance, you might feel a sense of guilt, especially if your spouse is going down this path with you reluctantly. After all, you have a child, so why can't you be satisfied? Why isn't this one child "enough"?

You also might feel like you're pushing your luck. Depending on the circumstances of how you had your first child, you might feel like it was a fluke. Maybe there won't be any birth parents choosing you this time. Maybe your eggs will be bad. Maybe there aren't any silver linings in your uterine lining this time, and the fertilized eggs won't take. The doubts run rampant.

While talking with friends and family might help, sometimes it hurts. They don't blame you for wanting to have a second child, but they might question you if you're working really hard at doing it. (This is another time you hear those oh-so-helpful "Just relax and you'll get pregnant!" comments. Ah, joy!) Whether you're going to the fertility clinic for early-morning blood work or jetting off to a foreign country's orphanage, you'll need support from others in caring for your child at home. You might worry that you're putting undo stress on your support system or your kid, and worry that it won't work, so the complications will all be for nothing in the end.

And maybe it won't work. But you won't know until you

194

try. But you're in a different place now. You're not childless, desperately hoping to become a parent. You are a parent. No matter how you got there, or how strange it sometimes feels to have finally arrived, you are parenting a child you love more than you thought possible. Your "baby hunger" may not be as desperate as the first time around. But then again, while you don't know *who* you're missing yet, you know what you're missing, since you're already a parent.

The desire to have another baby—not to mention give your much-loved child a sibling—can be just as painful as the first time around. But if you have problems getting another child, don't expect much sympathy from the "primary" infertile people. They might not say it aloud, but here's what they're thinking: "You've *got* a baby! How dare you complain about not having another one yet?" Admit it: When you were trying for baby number one, you may have thought the same thing about those with secondary infertility.

⌒ TIMING IS EVERYTHING

Almost as soon as I had [my first child], I was already in panic mode as to how we were going to have our next one, and if it was going to go OK—what I needed to do to start working on that. I nursed my son for about nine months and we went to the doctor probably when he was about six months old; we went back to the fertility clinic to talk about where I stood and what we were going to need to do for our next one, because I knew . . . I felt like I was in a race!

⌒MELISSA, 38 (TTC FOR 3 YEARS; 5-YEAR-OLD AND
2-YEAR-OLD SONS THROUGH FERTILITY TREATMENTS)

With your first child tucked tightly into your arms, you probably felt gratitude, relief, a sense of accomplishment. You made it. You did it. You finally did it! If you want one

195

child, or are undecided about your family's future size, another baby may not even be on the radar. But what if you know you want another baby before your incisions have healed? If you know you want to fill your arms with another child (and maybe another after that!), shouldn't you start now?

Time is a luxury that you might believe you just don't have. With your first child "under your belt," you now have the wisdom you need to pursue your dreams aggressively, so that you can continue with the business of being a parent.

Here's the conflict, however, one that is often unique to survivors of infertility. You know you need to get going with those adoption papers or fertility treatments, but you also want to focus your attention on your new baby—the one who's already here—and savor the moment. As you're rocking your baby back and forth in the glider, it strikes you that you feel a tad insane—and rocking back and forth is an appropriate activity for your current state of mind!

According to the National Center for Health Statistics, infertility impacts more than 3 million American women who already have had one or more successful pregnancies.

Feeling some resentment is expected and understandable. You worked so hard to have your child and now you can't fully relish the baby glow, since you need to go back to the salt mines of infertility. It's not fair that while you're a sleep-deprived zombie, you have worries weighing in the back of your mind about how you'll find another person to make you a sleep-deprived zombie!

Well, you've already learned from infertility that life isn't fair. As a bonus, you're a parent now, so you can multitask. You know your odds, and if you want to go for your second child, you understand that you need to get down to business and go for it. Experience has taught you that an adoption can take weeks—or years, and so can fertility treatments.

In the end, you might realize that diapers are a piece of cake compared to the despair you've felt from not having a baby in your arms. Just don't let your worries about the future detract from the amazing experience of becoming a parent for the first time. Your little person needs your focused attention.

⌒THE TREATMENT TOLL

> *When my son was six months old, we started trying for our second. The doctor said, "well, you've had one naturally, I'm sure you'll have one again." We're undergoing treatments and I feel bad, simply because I'm putting [my son] aside, and I don't even know if it's for a good reason.*

⌒DAWN, 36 (TTC FOR 3 YEARS; 3-YEAR-OLD SON
THROUGH FERTILITY TREATMENTS)

TIME FOR BIRTH CONTROL?

If you spent years desperately trying to get pregnant, taking birth control can make you feel like a fraud, wasting money for something that can't possibly happen. But, there's always that slim chance that lightning will strike. Right?

If your family is complete or if the chances of you conceiving pose a medical danger, there's no sense in using temporary birth control measures. Tying tubes or having a vasectomy can bring closure and peace of mind.

197

Deciding to start up again at a fertility clinic is a daunting proposition. If you left there euphoric, it may be dejecting to enter through the doors again. Your shoulders might drop; "Here we go again." On the other hand, you may feel more prepared for the ride. At least you've got someone in a car seat along with you.

If you sit in the waiting room with an infant in tow, you might feel as if you're imposing upon or even betraying your fellow patients or not as "qualified" to be there as others. Be sensitive. The woman sitting next to you may have just had her fourth unsuccessful round of IVF. She won't be entranced with your cooing baby. Remember how sensitive you were, before you got this little person? Get a sitter, or have a family member take care of your child while you go to your appointments.

The impact of treatment itself can also be physically challenging. The emotions, combined with hormonal changes, may cause depression, frustration, anger, bitterness—you name it! You remember those feelings, don't you?

But here's the difference. If you're emotional, those emotions can transfer to your child. If your child sees you cry, some of that stress might work its way into your child's life. And that may not be a price you're willing to pay. Depending on the age of their child, couples with secondary infertility must decide when and whether to tell the child about their struggles. For example, smaller children who see their mother taking shots or having blood drawn may become scared and wonder if she's sick. Older children might sense the stress in the family and wonder why they aren't enough to make their parents happy. That's a lot of guilt and worry for a little person to carry around.

So, keep in mind that if you talk about this with your

partner or anyone else, a kid over the age of twelve months is going to figure out something is going on. Your toddler may not know what's happening, but she knows that Mommy is crying all the time, or that Daddy is distracted. Think about the best approach to take with your kid(s), depending on age and maturity, to help him or her understand what's going on. Talking to children openly can be an opportunity to teach them that problems should be dealt with, not buried. And make sure that your kid knows that you love her more than anything—and that wanting another baby has nothing to do with some deficiency on her part.

multiple worries

Before your first child, the possibility that fertility treatments would result in having multiples seemed ideal. With an instant family, it's over and out for the fertility clinic and time to move on to the next phase in life.

When you're already a parent and enter through the clinic's doors for the second time around, though, the thought of having twins or more turns from joy into fear. You know how hard it is to take care of one baby, so the thought of two or more might be an unsettling prospect to you. Some studies estimate that your chance of having twins or more after fertility treatments is 1 in 38. Being an older mother also increases your chances for twins; if you're over forty-five, your chances increase by 17 percent. The chance (or "risk") of having higher order multiples (three or more babies) as a result of fertility treatments has soared over the last twenty years. The risk is real, so be prepared!

embies on the rocks

You're lucky. Your IVF round(s) was successful. You even have embryos left over. Just what do you do with those embryos waiting in the wings?

If you're trying again, you're probably relieved to have this backup. At least you're spared a month or two of "butt-shots" to stimulate your already abused ovaries, or it means you don't have to go through the egg donation route again. But if you're done having kids, what do you do with leftover embryos?

Do you abandon those "possible children" completely? After all, costs to store them add up—ranging from $200 to $1,000/year, and there's no guarantee that they'll ever "take." On the other hand, you know how hard you worked to create these possible kids. Depending on your religious or ethical beliefs, you may not be able to destroy them or have them used for research. Some couples choose to donate their embryos to other couples (sometimes called embryo adoption), but this is a decision that isn't for everyone. You might not want your children to have a sibling roaming around out there, somewhere. It's not just about you and your partner at this point. You must consider the feelings of your own child now. How does it impact them to know that they have full-blooded siblings?

This is a decision that may take weeks or months to resolve. Don't hesitate to talk to a qualified counselor as you determine the right choice for you and your family. The bottom line is that it's a private matter, and not anyone's business unless you tell people about it. Once you've decided how to handle the leftover embryos, you can decide if and what to tell people.

⌒ADOPTING THE SECOND TIME AROUND

Is my son going to be an only child? Until recently, I would have said yes. We lucked out with our adoption—we were chosen by our son's birth parents a couple of weeks after we were licensed, and they never wavered in their adoption decision. We became parents just six weeks later! We have an open adoption and we

200

love his birth parents and their families, and it's been such an amazing, positive experience for all of us, I worry that we won't be able to replicate that—or even come close.

And then there are the questions of time, money, relocating to a bigger house—everything you consider when you add another child to your family. The difference is that I'm not going to magically get pregnant and have the decision made for me—we have to do it ourselves one way or the other.

I debated for months, and it was stressful. Originally I'd wanted two kids, but Ryan was a terrible sleeper—he didn't sleep through the night until he was nineteen months old! I was so tired all the time, and I thought, screw it. I'll just be happy with one. I also felt guilty for wanting another child, when we have such an amazing, beautiful, wonderful little boy already. Shouldn't I be grateful for what I have?

Slowly I began to realize that I really wanted Ryan to grow up with a sibling. But I personally don't feel like that's enough of a reason to adopt again—it seems selfish to me. I thought about it, and talked to my husband about it, and prayed about it. Then one day, I realized, I really want another baby! I don't know where the feeling came from (maybe it was from finally sleeping again), but that was what I had been waiting for—the excitement, the anticipation, the joy. Now that we're opening our paperwork and I realize I'm going to be Mommy to another child, I'm thrilled! I know we probably won't have the "perfect" experience again—but that's not a reason to not have another child.

⌒KELLY, 41 (TTC FOR 6 YEARS; 2-YEAR-OLD SON
THROUGH DOMESTIC ADOPTION)

Like going through infertility treatments to pursue your second child, adoption is a conscious and deliberate decision. The decision to have more doesn't just fall on your lap. You have to put yourself out there and actively add to your family.

If you adopted your first child, you're a veteran of the process. You're wise to what home studies, adoption agencies, and lawyers are all about, and the paperwork you need to start. While you're at ease with the process part of the equation, you might be less confident that everything will come together as well as it did in the past. (Is it possible that all the stars can align again?)

Like before, you're excited—you're semi-expecting, after all! But you also have a fear that it might fall through. If you had a positive experience, you may worry that you won't be able to duplicate that. If you had a stressful experience the first time, or waited month after month to get the go-ahead to bring your child back to the United States, or had adoption matches fall through, you may worry that you can't get through it again. But hey, maybe this time you'll get lucky! This time will be a cinch! Or not. Obviously, there are no guarantees.

In some ways, you're more at ease and confident because you're already a parent. You're not going to flounder around with the car seat or feel awkward mixing formula. You know the drill. You don't have to showcase your natural ability with kids the way you did when you adopted for the first time. You're a parent now, and that's presumed.

But you're older now, too. Maybe that means you're less likely to be picked by a birth mom, or that you can't adopt from the same country again. Your available money to adopt may be less than last time—after all, you've got a kiddo and college fund to worry about already.

DOES ADOPTING A BABY "SOLVE" INFERTILITY?

We've all heard it before: So-and-so suffered through two (or twenty) years of infertility, adopted a baby, and then became pregnant two months later. In fact, studies have shown that pregnancy rates range from between only 3 percent to 10 percent post-adoption.

Adoption doesn't cure or jump-start infertility. More likely, for the 20 percent of infertile couples who have "unexplained infertility," the factors that contributed to being unable to conceive were somehow reduced. But if you do adopt, be prepared to hear these kinds of comments.

The most clueless and potentially hurtful comment? "Now that you've adopted, maybe you'll have a baby of your own!" Feel free to respond with a polite (or not-so-polite) version of, "We have a baby of our own—you're looking at him," and move on.

And you already have a child. What about the people who want to be parents but haven't adopted yet? Are you taking a child away from them? This is the adoptive parents' spin on secondary infertility. You may have many of the same emotions as parents going through fertility treatment to try again, which doesn't seem fair. Shouldn't you get a free pass, somehow?

Finally, you already have a child . . . to some, that's a disadvantage (this won't be your first child to dote on); to others, that's an advantage (you've ironed out the parenting kinks). If you participate in a domestic adoption, there's a good chance that your child's birth parents will have a say in whether you parent their babies or not. And out of birth moms who have a preference, about half choose families who don't have kids yet—they want their babies to be the first-born or only child. The other half want parents who have already have kids.

Because you have a child, you'll need to consider how much to tell him or her about the new child you're adding to your family. A child younger than two won't understand, but a three- or four-year-old may be delighted (or disgusted!) by the idea of becoming a big brother. Keep your child involved in the process, depending on age, and decide how much to share about how adoption works. Consider how you'll handle something going wrong, too, and make it clear that a placement that falls through, for example, could never happen with him or her.

The bottom line, though, as an adoptive parent is this—you hoped that the child you were meant to have would find you. And somehow he or she did. Now you must open your heart to another child by starting the process again—and believe that the next child will find you, too. Holding fast to that faith takes you from being the parent of one (or more) to the parent of two (or more).

⌒Caught Between Worlds

I would prefer not to be going through [infertility]. When your body fails you, it's really frustrating. Especially now that I have one, you get caught between two worlds—you're not really infertile because you have a child, but you are because you can't have another and you still have the mentality of being infertile even though you have one. You're stuck in the middle.

⌒Jennifer, 37 (TTC for 3 years; 2-year-old daughter through fertility treatments)

When you were trying to get pregnant the first time, you found that the old adage "misery loves company" couldn't be truer. Maybe you reached out to support groups, finding the camaraderie uplifting. If you were more private about your struggles, you may have glued your attention to online message boards and chat sessions, where you could pour your heart out to an understanding and compassionate audience.

When you finally found yourself in the lucky position of being pregnant or on the verge of adopting, though, you may have suddenly felt like an outcast. In fact, many organizations and web sites have explicit rules on what you can and cannot share when it comes to children, so that the feelings of the continuing infertile people are protected.

Then, when you finally became a parent, you felt as if you'd betrayed your infertile friends and had to choose your words carefully when you were around them. For example, you couldn't complain about feeling strung out by your previous seven sleepless nights . . . because you know they would give anything to have seven hundred of those.

So, it was time to find a new group for support. That group of moms who meet for coffee around the corner shared sound advice about babyproofing the house and were sometimes more than forthcoming on what sex is like after having a baby. You found camaraderie again. But then, as if on cue, this group started becoming pregnant with their second babies, and you started your infertility cycles again. You might feel alienated.

Unlike those with primary infertility, these couples don't receive much pity. "I'd have more sympathy for you if you didn't already have your son," is a phrase people will think—and some will even utter. Like we said earlier, "primaries" themselves may not have any empathy as well, so be forewarned. Try to remember how it felt when you didn't know if you would ever "make it" and become a parent, and cut them some slack.

Another unique challenge for secondary infertility patients is that they must be part of the parent scene daily. Hearing others talking about how easily they conceived or complaining about being pregnant can sometimes be too much to bear.

As a result, you might start avoiding certain groups or parenting situations so that you can shield yourself from the pregnancy talk. If it serves as a constant reminder that you're unable to conceive, you might be better off taking a break and making some new friends.

⌒FEELING AT PEACE WITH YOUR FAMILY'S SIZE

If you're struggling with secondary infertility, it might be a smart move for your mental health to put a time frame on your efforts. Just as you did the first time around, a grand plan will start to make you feel more in control, but also more accepting of the outcome, however it turns out.

Recognize also that even if you started your family with a bang of multiples, it still might give you pause when you contemplate whether or not you should try to pull up another chair to the kitchen table. Yours might be a noisy house, but there still might be a feeling in your heart that someone is missing. "Regular" families go through the same thing, and there are no easy answers to know if your family is the "right" size.

Whether the feelings of absence are due to infertility or are simply part of coming to terms with your own mortality, try to focus on the people who matter most: the ones who are with you now. If you don't, you may regret the lost times later.

THE BELATED BABY

10

Infertile Forever:
YOUR JOURNEY AS A PARENT AND AS A PERSON

[Infertility] has deepened me. For example, I think I have always been a compassionate person, but infertility has made me have even more compassion for people. With few exceptions, we are all extremely grateful for our children, but I think I have an even deeper level of gratitude than I would have had they come more easily.

As far as how adoption has changed me, it feels like my heart has just been opened up wider. To have a complete stranger handed to you and to be told you are now his parents, and have that child accept you so readily, and for you to just dive in and start loving and parenting that child and accept him as what he now is, "your own," is an experience that just forever changes you.

—JULIE, 49 (TTC FOR 3 YEARS; 7-YEAR-OLD SON THROUGH INTERNATIONAL ADOPTION AND 3-YEAR-OLD "SURPRISE" SON)

All you wanted was a baby.

In the end, that's exactly what you got—plus a whole lot more than you bargained for! You got the ride of your life on the proverbial "infertility rollercoaster," and lo and behold, you weren't thrown off.

For the first time in your life, you learned that sometimes no matter how hard you try—how well you take care of yourself, how many books you read or what types of medications you swallow—you don't always get what you want . . . or at least what you want right when you want it. Your bewilderment at this stark fact may have led to depression and difficulties with your spouse. You rejected those who love you the most but didn't know how to help. Bitterness ruled. Money was lost, and so was time.

Ironically, whether you have one child or are surrounded by many, you can still feel "infertile" at times. You've sunk to the lowest of lows and, like a war veteran, you'll never forget how awful and empty that felt. You'd lost control over your future, and you now realize that you never had any to begin with. There were ultimately bigger plans—and people—in store for you. You now can't imagine living life without those plans unfolding as they did!

All of those months or years spent in complete frustration, sadness, and fear gave you not only a child, but also a character that won't quit. When you carefully pick apart the entire experience, you'll begin to recognize the benefits of having been barren: You have a stronger union with your spouse; you have more empathy for others; you're more patient with people than you ever were before.

Some of God's greatest gifts are unanswered prayers.

⌐Garth Brooks

Gee, gaining more love, kindness, and patience for others—sounds like a good foundation for successful parenting, doesn't it?

The truth is that no one escapes infertility unscathed. It can leave you feeling bitter, angry, spiteful, desolate, and brokenhearted. But it can also make you a better parent—more sensitive, more appreciative, and yes, more grateful.

208

THE BELATED BABY

⌒ TAKEAWAY LESSONS

The challenge of infertility was one of the greatest challenges of your life—possibly the biggest challenge. It forced you to cope and to make a plan. It cajoled your character to grow when all you wanted to do was shrivel up in a corner and die.

When you were struggling to keep yourself together as you did everything you could to become a parent, you probably didn't stop and analyze what you were learning. In fact, you couldn't have cared less about that! All you knew was that you wanted complete, utter, and permanent resolution in the form of a bundle of joy in a bassinet, which would give you an off ramp from your insane infertility "journey."

The only thing you wanted was a baby, but you were rewarded with so much more.

profound gratefulness

> There's not a day that goes by that I don't feel completely lucky and blessed that [I got pregnant and had a daughter]. And again, I don't know if it had happened naturally if I would think it every single day. Of course, I would still love my kid, but would I take it for granted? I wonder that sometimes.
>
> ⌒KATHLEEN, 42 (TTC FOR 3 YEARS; 1-YEAR-OLD
> DAUGHTER THROUGH FERTILITY TREATMENTS)

Did you ever think infertility was God's way of punishing you for something you'd done in your deep dark past? Maybe you found yourself asking questions such as "why me?" and "what did I do to deserve this?" Deep down you may even still carry these questions around in your heart, and worry that karma somehow caught up with you and that's why you had to suffer so much to become a mom or

209

dad. Logically, though, you know those thoughts are unfounded and probably now often forget that you even had them!

Rather than dwelling on why infertility happened to you, you're now in a position to be able to see clearly what the experience *gave* to you. Maybe you realize that you had felt entitled to have children, right when you wanted to have them. And now you realize what a gift they are and how much joy they add to your life.

Hopefully, even if you're still anguishing to add more children to your family, you can focus on the meaning-packed, everyday moments and milestones with your child. Her first belly laugh. The first day of preschool. A tap dance recital that's excruciatingly long . . . and loud. Slow down and zero in on these simple times; the reality is, they are the best of times and will be gone tomorrow.

Feeling thankful, blessed, and lucky is the only way all parents should feel—on the majority of days at least! Be glad that for you, infertility has maybe shined an extra bit of bright light on those feelings.

deeper sense of empathy

> Five years is a huge part of your adult life . . . the whole experience of what I learned from [infertility] and who I am is impacted by it. When I see people who have kids or who are pregnant, my mind automatically goes to, "I wonder if this was an easy time of life for them, or if they had a struggle with this like I did . . ." I wonder if they're okay and how this all impacted their life. [Those of us who've been infertile] are sort of like a family; we have this connection.
>
> ⌒Melissa, 38 (TTC for 5 years; 5-year-old and 2-year-old sons through fertility treatments)

THE BELATED BABY

Before you even had an inkling that you'd be starting your own family, you may have been the brash one asking couples when they were going to start theirs. "You'd make great parents!" you might have cheered or nagged, "so, when are you going to get busy and get pregnant?" You made those comments before the infertility bug struck you, though, and now you cringe that they ever left your lips. Now you're most likely pretty cautious when it comes to probing people about their plans. If you sense that there might be something wrong, you know that being mute is the sensitive move—that is until the person asks you for your side of the story.

Consider how your newfound gentle spirit has had a ripple effect to other areas in your relationships with others. Or not! You may be just as feisty as ever. But you probably have more empathy for all types of other life situations now, because you understand that there are motives behind why people behave the way they do. For example, you know that your friend Jeanie isn't going with you to the zoo because she just had a miscarriage and can't face being around a bunch of kids. Your cousin can't make the reunion because he's just had a relapse of cancer. Whether you're a little easier on a spaced-out waitress or renew a relationship with an estranged friend, infertility can yield some unexpected positive benefits.

more patience

[Due to infertility] I'm definitely more patient. Part of that could be that it took longer for me to be a mom and I'm just older. Older people have been through more experiences in life in general, so that kind of gives you some wisdom. Again, my gratitude is just so big, I just

feel happy every time I see [my daughter], just so happy.

ꝏKim, 44 (TTC for 5 years; 4-year-old daughter through fertility treatments and gestational surrogate)

You can look at [infertility] in a positive way. I don't think we let the normal stressors that face new parents bother us—I think we were actually able to handle them a little bit better, because we were just so grateful that we had our son. So I think we took less for granted. I don't think we were bothered by the small stuff. We were really prepared by the time that he came along, so I think we were pretty mature about it. We weren't as frazzled as some of our friends, just because we were just so friggin' lucky to have this kid.

ꝏTracy, 35 (TTC for 3 years; 3-year-old and 7-month-old sons through fertility treatments)

I'm a more relaxed mother, and I wouldn't have been if I hadn't gone through this. My very close friends are surprised at how laid back of a mother I am, because normally I'm very high-strung, like high control freak kind of person. But as a mother, I'm very laid back, relaxed; my kids are very happy and relaxed as a result of it. I think that's partly a result of having gone through what we did and having that, worrying about everything— but now just being happy to have two little kids, who you know, if they're both screaming at the same time, it's going to stop in a few minutes. Try and not get too worked up about things like that that are temporary.

ꝏLisa, 33 (TTC for 2 years; newborn boy/girl twins through fertility treatments)

Do you smile inwardly when others stress about how stressed out their kids are making them? You recognize better than most that a tantrum by a two-year-old is temporary, and that dirt under fingernails can always come clean.

What's made you so grounded despite the inevitable chaos that kids bring to your life is the fact that you know how close you were to them never being part of your life. Your family is the direct result of your hard work and determination despite the odds against you. Had you chosen a different path—i.e., abandoning the pursuit of a baby altogether to live a "child free" existence—you would never have had the opportunity to endlessly empty the dishwasher or rock a child in the middle of the night to comfort his growing pains.

You have the gift of insight on the alternatives of your current life. Chances are this knowledge gives you patience to deal with the small stuff.

return of faith

> I'm not a super religious person, but I really became a very spiritual person. [Infertility] made me have faith. I had faith someone good was going to happen to me, whoever that might be. Is it going to be an adopted baby, is the IVF going to work . . . at some point, you just have to take a leap of faith, and I really believe that if you just hang in there and have faith and are positive, and get in touch with that spiritual side, good things, a good outcome will come.
>
> ᗡMARISA, 37 (TTC FOR 4 YEARS; 2-YEAR-OLD BOY/GIRL
> TWINS THROUGH FERTILITY TREATMENTS)

> I don't check for breathing anymore these days, but, you know, making sure they're fine, I still do that. Every night, I will check. Basically, having to say to God, OK, you gave me this perfect baby, and I went through so much to have her, and then I finally had to say, OK, I

213

don't want to be this neurotic crazy mother, so I'm going to put my faith in you again . . . that you're going to take care of this child for me, so I'm not a neurotic mother. But I do find that when they're sick, like if they're sick and spiking a really high fever . . . that old fertility thing kind of sneaks up on me.

~KAREN, 47 (TTC FOR 6 YEARS; 13-YEAR-OLD DAUGHTER AND
9-YEAR-OLD TWIN SONS THROUGH FERTILITY TREATMENTS)

As sad as [having breast cancer was], I can tell you that I've never been happier and the cancer has brought me a lot of grace and beauty. I'm really grateful for life, and my health, and every day is such a blessing. I can look at infertility and breast cancer now as lessons in inspiration. They've given me great life lessons. You have to be okay with question marks.

~KIM, 44 (TTC FOR 5 YEARS; 4-YEAR-OLD DAUGHTER
THROUGH FERTILITY TREATMENTS AND GESTATIONAL SURROGATE)

Instead of ruminating on why God punished you, as you may have done during infertility, you may discover that in the end, God was rewarding you. During your struggles, you may have held strong to the belief that you would be connected with the child who was meant for you all along, somehow. And at last, you were! As a result, your faith may have deepened throughout the process of infertility, whether that means you're a faithful follower of the Baptist church or simply more spiritual in general, and you take time to enjoy the beauty inherent in everyday life.

Infertility taught you all about control . . . when you could have it, and when you needed to let it go. It was an excruciating process and painful moment when you realized that you had no power over your own destiny—and you now know for certain that you never will.

214

THE SERENITY PRAYER

Did you memorize and repeat the serenity prayer a thousand times during infertility? Wait a minute—it comes in quite handy for parenting, too!

"God, give us grace to accept with serenity the things that cannot be changed, courage to change the things that should be changed, and the wisdom to distinguish the one from the other."

REINHOLD NIEBUHR, THEOLOGIAN (1892–1971)

Relish the fact that your wisdom about control makes you that much better prepared for parenting. While you no doubt influence what type of person your child becomes and the values he carries, you ultimately have zero control over his unique and fundamental personality. Whether he's shy and thoughtful or as rambunctious as they come, you must accept him for who he is. For example, while you can force him to have manners, you can't control his likes and dislikes, or when he'll choose to use the potty. No matter how he came into your life, he is his own miracle and his own person.

☞ THICKER SKIN

My husband had open heart surgery last year. And he's fine; it was a congenital problem but involved some very serious surgery. I kept thinking "yeah, I'm a strong cookie, I can deal with it." But my infertility experience really, really helped me cope with the whole thing. I'm not intimidated by physicians, I know what kind of questions to ask, and I know how to deal with them.

215

I'm a stronger person. I think that any challenge in life makes you stronger; it's not always the easy things in life, it's how you deal with the challenges.

♥KAREN, 47 (TTC FOR 6 YEARS; 13-YEAR-OLD DAUGHTER AND 9-YEAR-OLD TWIN SONS THROUGH FERTILITY TREATMENTS)

Did being infertile help you grow a spine? In dealing with adoption lawyers, doctors, nurses, and insensitive family members, you may have needed to be more forceful and say things that were atypical of your personality type. Unfortunately, sometimes you need to demand an appointment or tell an acquaintance to "buzz off" in order to stick up for yourself.

Think through the times when you had to step up and speak up. A parent-in-perpetual-waiting can be a force to be reckoned with, and you probably surprised others—and yourself!—by the depth of your assertiveness. You studied and planned a course of action. Now that you know how to navigate the systems of fertility clinics and adoption agencies, look out—there's no holding you back for what will inevitably come your way in the future.

Recognize and validate in your own mind that infertility was a life or death crisis. You know that you CAN mourn someone who hasn't been born, and someone you were never given the chance to meet. You've grieved, and you've grown.

If infertility was the only tough life card you were dealt, you'd be pretty lucky, wouldn't you? But as you know, the future is filled with just as much uncertainty as you felt during that time in your life. Aging parents will need living assistance or have medical problems. Disease will strike. Jobs will be lost. But you're prepared. You've been tested by a life crisis and survived. You're positioned to apply the strength that infertility gave you.

216

broadened horizons

Adopting internationally has expanded my mind to include a more global way of thinking. Whereas the picture in my mind of "my world" might have looked like a map of the U.S., that same mental image now includes a much larger part of the world that includes the part from which we found our son.

〜JULIE, 49 (TTC FOR 3 YEARS; 7-YEAR-OLD SON THROUGH INTERNATIONAL ADOPTION AND 3-YEAR-OLD "SURPRISE" SON)

Whether you're a travel buff or would rather sit home on the couch with a movie and popcorn, if your infertility trip included a trip to a non-U.S. destination to adopt your child, chances are that it rocked you to the core. You saw things that you will never be able to "unsee." You witnessed people living in destitute, impoverished situations. Hunger and substandard living conditions were the norm. You're not ashamed to say that you're glad you never have to return, at least not for a while.

Turn your wounds into wisdom.

〜OPRAH WINFREY

When you return home to overhear moms in line at preschool complaining about the long lines at Target, you'll recall the children you met at an orphanage lining up for a meal. They'd be happy with half of the things we buy and take for granted.

Your child serves as a forever reminder of the country and culture from which he came from. It's a humbling and honorable position to be his parent. You'll always know that even though your family comes first, there's also and always a bigger picture.

ᏩPARENTS, WITH PLENTY OF PRACTICE!

As hard as it was, the worst years of my life, and as painful as it was, I would not go back and change it, because I do think I'm definitely a stronger person. Our marriage is stronger, I'm probably a better mother. I don't know better; I'm different, I don't think I'd go back and change it at all.

ᏩLISA, 33, (TTC FOR 4 YEARS; MOM TO 1-YEAR-OLD TWINS
THROUGH FERTILITY TREATMENTS)

Remember when it was popular to put an item on layaway? Maybe your mom pined for a ruby red coat hanging in the department store window, so the manager tucked it away in the back of the store for her. Then, she paid for the object of her affection each payday by payday, until at last she earned the right to drape it over her shoulders and wear it proudly. (Was the coat warmer than it would have been if she had used her credit card? Did it feel more luxurious? Was she more worried about coffee spilling on it?)

Those who've hit the baby jackpot on "month one" are a little like those who make an impulsive credit card purchase: They knew they wanted it and they received immediate gratification, but they may not have had time to come to terms emotionally with what they'd done. It doesn't mean they didn't want a baby just as much as the layaway folks. They just didn't spend as much time fantasizing about how wonderful being a parent would be, and how spectacular a privilege it is to be one.

You, on the other hand, had to wait in the layaway line, and had to scrape together enough money, energy, and hope every month in order to "earn" the object of your desires. Of course, there wasn't an official time that the layaway came due. The uncertainty in that bleak fact almost

THE BELATED BABY

drove you crazy. You had to trust in a higher power that it would happen, which it finally has.

Don't discount the fact that in many ways, you assumed the role of "parent" long before you ever became one. You made a conscious choice to become a mom or a dad, unlike someone whose egg and sperm "miraculously" collided one night and created another human being. Unlike them, you had the benefit of time (sometimes too much of it, thank you very much!) to ponder what kind of parent you wanted to be and how you wanted to raise your family.

> *The world breaks everyone and afterwards, many are strong at the broken places.*
>
> ᗉ‍ERNEST HEMINGWAY
> (1899–1961)

You're older, wiser, and better prepared for the parenting panics that will inevitably come your way. Just as you didn't expect or want to be tested by infertility, you'll find the same challenges will come to you in parenting. From your toddler tripping and chipping his two front teeth on a tiled floor to your high school senior being despondent that she didn't get into her first college of choice, there's never a dull moment.

The ride of life continues—and thank goodness it includes a child now!

experts in sacrifice

> *The people who don't experience problems and the frustrations of trying to get pregnant, they truly . . . I don't want to say they take it for granted, but it's really just hard for them to relate and understand, because there are a lot of sacrifices that you have to make to try to get those little ones.*

> ᗉ‍GREG, 36 (TTC FOR 6 YEARS; BIOLOGICAL
> 1-YEAR-OLD TWIN SONS)

219

Going through infertility is similar to an early form of parenting: You've had to make sacrifices before wailing cries ever entered through your front door. To begin with, when you add up the amount of time you spent driving to and from clinics, researching your options and reading books about fertility and adoption, you realize that it was probably equal to (or greater than!) at least a part-time job. And rather than receive a supplemental income for that job, you had to pay thousands of dollars in medical bills and adoption fees. In addition to time and money, you sacrificed your body.

You're perfectly prepared for parenthood, because this kid has been cramping your style since long before he even hit the scene! For many, the transition to parenting is difficult if they've always put their needs in the number one position. Whether it was two golf games a day or shopping sprees that never stopped, habits can be hard to break just because a baby is born. You, however, have had early practice in surrendering your past pleasures. It's no big deal for you to spend quiet evenings "in" to be with your family; quite the opposite—it's a privilege to do so.

does infertility make better parents?

It sounds snotty, but I really feel like people who go through any kind of struggle to build their family [are] a little bit better parents. Most people won't want to hear that. Maybe it's just that we have such a deeper appreciation and that we grasp the miracle and the joy more than someone who just said, "Oh, I want to have my baby in June, so I'm going to conceive in September."

We're more appreciative, more patient. We can find joy in everything, and not just the good things.

⌒Anita, 43 (TTC for 4 years; 7-year-old twin sons through fertility treatments and donor egg)

THE BELATED BABY

I know this will probably piss off everybody who hasn't gone through infertility—it's a group no one wants to be part of—but I just feel more appreciative. I don't take my parenting for granted. And I'm not insinuating anybody else does by any means. But my husband and I go into [our son's] room every night before he goes to bed and we have this ritual where we put him to bed together. As he's drifting off, we both just stand there in his room watching him. I bet you four out of seven nights a week I'm sitting there crying just looking at my son. I just feel so fortunate and blessed to have him in my life.

> ☞Heather, 32 (TTC for 3 years; 1-year-old son through fertility treatments)

I wonder every day if I really do love my kids just a little more than anyone else loves their kids. Isn't that crazy? In my mind I know everybody (or almost everybody) feels that way about their own kids. But somewhere in my smug little mind or my overflowing heart, I can't believe others really do. I can't believe anyone else can feel this way, too.

Maybe that is the ultimate gift of infertility for those lucky enough to end up as a parent, in whatever way . . . maybe we love just a little bit more.

> ☞Patti, 42 (TTC for 5 years; 5-year-old son and 3-year-old daughter through infertility treatments)

Ah yes, you've gained so much empathy and compassion for others through infertility, and that's why now you're going to come right out and say it: You're a better parent than those who didn't experience a day of infertility! (Be honest. Do you ever feel this way, even just a little?) Maybe some days you do. After all, you felt inferior to all

221

of the fertile people in the world for so long, maybe now you just have an urge to showcase a superiority complex on occasion. There must be a badge of honor lurking somewhere from the experience, right? Did you earn the right to gloat . . . just a little bit?

all you need is love

The truth is that no one's cornered the market on love. No other person can measure the contents of someone else's heart or judge how deeply they care. And of course, no one is perfect, either. Just because you worked extra hard to have your kids doesn't mean you won't blow your top when they are unruly.

A mother's love for her child is like nothing else in the world.

⌐AGATHA CHRISTIE
(1890–1976)

In fact, the farther away you drift from infertility, the more immersed in "normal" parenting you will become. As time passes, the sting of infertility will lessen. But you'll always know that the worst day of parenting is always infinitely better than your best day during infertility.

All you wanted was a baby. But what you received was so much more.

Now that you have your beloved, belated baby, you are stronger, wiser, and filled with more love than you ever thought possible.

Congratulations.

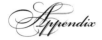

Organizations/Online Resources

The American Fertility Association

305 Madison Avenue Suite 449

New York, NY 10165

E-mail: info@theafa.org

(888) 917–3777

www.theafa.org

Founded in 1999, the AFA works to transform the lives of couples facing infertility, raise awareness of and education about reproductive diseases, and fight for social and legislative changes.

American Society for Reproductive Medicine (ASRM)

1209 Montgomery Highway

Birmingham, AL 35216–2809

E-mail: asrm@asrm.org

(205) 978–5000

www.asrm.org

Nonprofit leader in providing multidisciplinary information, education, advocacy, and standards in the field of reproductive medicine.

223

RESOLVE: The National Infertility Association

8405 Greensboro Drive, Suite 800

McLean, VA 22102–5120

(703) 556–7172

www.resolve.org

Since 1974, RESOLVE offers national support through a network of regional and local chapters.

The InterNational Council on Infertility Information Dissemination, Inc. (INCIID)

P.O. Box 6836

Arlington, VA 22206

(703) 379–9178

www.inciid.org

INCIID helps individuals and couples by providing immediate information about and support for infertility treatment and guidance on other family-building options. The parenting message boards offer specific support to those who have given birth, have multiples, or adopted after infertility.

Parenting and Infertility Websites

www.adopt.org: The website for the National Adoption Center expands opportunities for children in foster care by showing photo profiles of those kids waiting to be adopted. It also provides information about adoption and an "adoption clubhouse," for kids ages eight to thirteen who've been adopted and their families.

www.adoptivefamilies.com: This is a comprehensive resource for parents with adopted children—they offer web-only content from their magazine of the same name, along with "quick links" to domestic as well as international adoption information. You'll also find adoption stories from other parents.

www.babble.com/babblepedia: On this collaborative website, you can swap your best parenting secrets with other parents.

www.belatedbaby.com: The official website for this book. Learn more about the authors, buy a t-shirt to raise money for and awareness about infertility, and share your story of how infertility has impacted your parenting experience.

www.breastfeeding.com: Visit the "Buddy Boutique" for nursing bras and other clothing designed for nursing mothers. The site also has a national directory of lactation consultants, along with Q&A forums that address issues involving breastfeeding in public, choosing the right breast pump for you, and other related topics.

www.breastfeedingavenue.com: This site includes breastfeeding tips, an online store, and a list of resources for nursing moms.

www.breastfeedingonline.com: If you've adopted a child and want to breastfeed, check out this site, which is filled with resources and articles all about adoptive breastfeeding. It includes videos on breastfeeding and online pamphlets on various topics regarding nursing.

www.cafemom.com: If you're the mother of an adoptive child, this is the place for you. After registering for free, join one of the many groups ranging from foster parenting to international adoption. Also, you can post pictures of your family and read online journals of other parents in addition to posting your own.

www.caringbridge.com: Create your own free, personalized website to share information with family and friends during a time of crisis, such as critical illness, treatment, or recovery.

www.donorsiblingregistry.com: The Donor Sibling Registry helps people who were conceived through sperm, egg, or embryo donation locate those with whom they have genetic ties.

www.thefamilycorner.com: This website has various experts online to answer questions, ranging from medical concerns to gardening. They offer tips on frugal living, crafts, and fun activities to do with the kids. Take advantage of their free newsletter and forums as well.

www.thefamilypost.com: Share your family photos and videos online, but not with the world. Create your own professional looking website and post in a secure environment.

www.fathersworld.com: A unique website that is tailored to fathers, complete with an online DVD/bookstore with useful resources just for dads.

www.iparenting.com: An extremely comprehensive website, this resource has nearly everything a parent could want—a free e-newsletter, blogs, links to other parenting sites, a "tech center," as well as expert Q & A, a more recent addition to the site.

www.ivillage.com: While this is not a parenting-specific website, it offers tons of information under its "Pregnancy and Parenting" category. Check out the resources for "older" parents, like a message board for parents in their forties and fifties.

www.kellymom.com: This site has a store that sells books and nursing supplies; it also has forums for nursing mothers, as well as polls and surveys about the benefits of breastfeeding.

www.lalecheleague.org: This helpful resource offers new mothers an online store with breastfeeding books, links to your legal breastfeeding rights, an event calendar, and forums and podcasts to assist with all of your needs. La Leche League is bilingual as well, offering resources for Spanish-speaking women.

www.momspace.com: Designed to save moms time and money, MomSpace gives you information you need about local businesses and connects you with other moms in your area.

226

www.mops.org: Mothers of Preschoolers, unite! This Christian organization brings mothers of children together to build friendships, exchange parenting strategies, and meet mentors.

www.nomotc.org: The National Organization of Mothers of Twins Club, Inc., website offers information to parents of multiples, from twins on up, and connects parents with clubs for personal support.

www.parenthood.com: You'll find lots of parenting-related resources including discussion boards, polls and surveys, and a comprehensive A-Z topics list.

www.parentzone.com: This free website offers loads of helpful extras, like a weekly newsletter; finance, health, and fitness tips; and message boards for parents.

www.pluggedinparent.com: Worried about how your kids use technology and how to keep track of it? Plug yourself into this website for tips.

www.surrogacy.com: This site offers a way for donors and recipients to connect with one another through classified ads, and offers message boards, too.

www.surromomsonline.com: This homespun site provides information, support, and personal stories to people interested in pursuing a surrogacy or egg/sperm donor arrangement, as well as comprehensive and active message boards for connecting with others.

www.tripletconnection.org: The Triplet Connection offers publications as well as extensive online support for families with higher order multiples.

www.yoga4fertility.com: For those going through secondary infertility, check out Brenda Strong's website on how to enhance and support your fertility protocol by practicing yoga, either solo or with your partner.

Books for Parents

Adopting After Infertility. Patricia Irwin Johnston (Perspectives Press, 1992). This book is for adoptive parents who are infertile. It is broken into three basic sections: the challenge of infertility, making the commitment to adoption, and adoption through a lifetime. It covers the adoption process and how to choose between different types of adoption (i.e., domestic versus international).

Attaching in Adoption: Practical Tools for Today's Parents. Deborah D. Gray (Perspectives Press, 2002). Therapist and author Gray writes a comprehensive parenting manual to describe children who are challenged in attachment due to neglect, grief, abuse, and prenatal exposure to addictive substances.

The Baby Business: How Money, Science, and Politics Drive the Commerce of Conception. Debora L. Spar (Harvard Business School Press, 2006). This book examines fertility treatment from a business perspective, exploring some of the ethical, financial, and practical issues surrounding ART, or assisted reproductive technology—which is a $3 billion industry.

Twenty Things Adopted Kids Wish Their Adoptive Parents Knew. Sherrie Eldridge (Delta, 1999). This book offers full coverage of the emotional and communication issues involved in adoption from the author, who herself was adopted.

Toddler Adoption: The Weaver's Craft. Mary Hopkins-Best (Perspectives Press, 1997). This book serves as a complete guide for anyone who adopts a toddler. It covers the transition period into the home and first impressions, as well as detailed strategies for achieving a positive attachment.

APPENDIX

What Size Shoe Does She Wear? Adopting a Toddler. Denise Harris
Hoppenhauer (iUniverse Star, 2002). An adoptive mom of two
children from Russia, Hoppenhauer writes a nuts-and-bolts
guide to bringing your child home, from wardrobe ideas to
childproofing tips.

CHILDREN'S BOOKS

*All About Adoption: How Families Are Made and How Kids Feel
About It.* Marc A. Nemiroff and Jane Annunziata, illustrated by
Carol Koeller (Imagination Press, 2003). A book for older children and their parents on the intricacies of emotions involved
with adoption. Written by clinical psychologists.

The Day We Met You. Phoebe Koehler (Aladdin Picture Books,
1997). Adoptive parents describe how they prepared for the
arrival of their new baby in this heartwarming picture book.

The Family Book. Todd Parr (Little, Brown Young Readers, 2003).
Teaches young children about the variety of families that exist,
and that although we're all different, we all love the same way.

*The Kangaroo Pouch: A Story About Gestational Surrogacy for Young
Children.* Sarah Phillips Pellet, illustrated by Laurie A. Faust
(Trafford Publishing, 2007). A picture book for small children
to introduce the concept of surrogacy and the decisions and
process involved.

If Kisses Were Colors. Janet Lawler, illustrated by Alison Jay (Dial,
2003). A picture book that depicts the endless depth of a parent's love for her child.

A Mother for Choco . Keiko Kasza (Putnam Juvenile, 1996). A picture book that proves families are created not by looks, but by
love.

Over the Moon: An Adoption Tale. Karen Katz (Henry Holt, 1997).
Excellent picture book, especially for those families built
through Chinese adoption.

Tell Me Again about the Night I Was Born. Jamie Lee Curtis (Joanna Cotler, 1996). Sweet, humorous, and lively book about adoption.

We Belong Together. (Little, Brown Young Readers, 2007). A book just for adoptive families of all kinds; celebrates and recognizes how special adoption is.

APPENDIX

Glossary

401(k): Employer-sponsored retirement plan named after the section of the Internal Revenue Code that created it.

Adoptive breastfeeding: Process where adoptive mothers stimulate milk production so they can nurse their adopted child(ren).

Amniocentesis: Medical test performed between 15 and 18 weeks of pregnancy that identifies some of the fetus' genetic risk factors by examining amniotic fluid extracted from the uterus.

ART (assisted reproductive technologies): Can refer to any type of treatment to aid conception but usually refers to in vitro fertilization ("IVF") and embryo transfer.

BFP++++ (big fat positive): Acronym used (often in online forums and chat rooms) to refer to positive pregnancy test results.

Birth parent(s): The biological mother and/or father of a child placed for adoption.

Chemical pregnancy: Refers to an early miscarriage or the failure of a fertilized egg to implant in the uterus.

Clomid: Clomiphene citrate, an oral fertility drug used to induce ovulation.

Closed adoption: An adoption where there is no contact information exchanged between adoptive and birth parents, and/or no contact occurs between birth and adoptive parents after the child is placed with the adoptive parents.

C-section (Caesarean section): When a baby is delivered through a surgical incision made in the mother's abdomen and uterus as opposed to a vaginal delivery. While some C-sections are elective, they may also be performed when the life of the mother or baby is at risk.

CVS (chorionic villus sampling): Medical test performed at 10 to 13 weeks of pregnancy that identifies some of the fetus' genetic risk factors.

D&C (dilation and curettage): Medical procedure which stands for dilation, or opening the entrance of a woman's uterus, and curettage, which means scraping. A D&C is often performed after a miscarriage to ensure that no tissue remains inside the woman's uterus.

Domestic adoption: An adoption involving a child born and adopted within the United States. It may be private, also called "independent," or an agency adoption where adoptive parents work with an adoption agency. The laws of the state where the adoptive parents reside (and sometimes where the baby or child resides) control the adoption process.

Donor eggs: Eggs used to create an embryo that are not from the mother of the child; they can be donated by a friend, relative, or stranger. (Women's egg quality tends to decline as they get older, so they may use donor eggs to become pregnant.)

Donor sperm: Sperm used to create an embryo that is not from the father of the child.

232

E2 (estradiol): A female hormone that rises during pregnancy; E2 levels are usually monitored during ART.

Ectopic: Usually refers to an ectopic pregnancy, when a fertilized egg implants in a fallopian tube or location other than the uterus. It's a life-threatening condition for the mother.

Embryo adoption option: People who have completed fertility treatment but have "left-over" embryos sometimes allow others to "adopt" their embryos to become pregnant.

EPT: Early pregnancy test.

Exclusive breastfeeding: Refers to a mother feeding her baby breast milk only (i.e., no formula or other liquids or foods) for her baby's first six months of life.

Freeze some eggs: The process of having eggs retrieved and stored to use to attempt pregnancy at a later date; some women are choosing to "save" eggs for when they want to become pregnant.

FSH (follicle-stimulating hormone): Hormone that stimulates the production of egg(s) in women; its levels are monitored during fertility treatment.

Gestational surrogate: When one woman serves as the "host" uterus to another woman's biological embryo. For this type of arrangement, legal, financial, and counseling considerations must be made, even if the surrogate is a friend or family member.

Gestational diabetes: A condition that occurs when a pregnant woman's body can't make enough insulin and glucose builds to high levels. It affects about 4 percent of all pregnant women, putting babies at risk for developing obesity, breathing problems, and diabetes.

HCG (human chorionic gonadotropin): Hormone injection that stimulates egg production during fertility treatments.

ICSI (intracytoplasmic sperm injection): The process of injecting a single sperm directly into a mature egg with a glass needle.

International adoption: Adoption by U.S. citizens involving a child born outside the United States and usually facilitated through an agency. The laws of the country where the child is born/resides control the adoption process.

IRA (Individual Retirement Account): Special retirement account allowed by the IRS to provide tax-deferred contributions or growth; a way to supplement other forms of retirement savings.

IRL (in real life): Term used online to describe personally known, "offline" friends, versus those friendships formed on the Internet.

IUI (intra-uterine insemination): The process of injecting sperm through a catheter directly into the cervix to raise the odds of fertilization.

IVF (in-vitro fertilization): The process of placing sperm and an unfertilized egg together in a Petri dish to achieve fertilization; fertilized eggs that survive to three or five days are then transferred back into a woman's uterus to achieve pregnancy.

Miscarriage: The loss of a pregnancy. It's estimated that 25 percent of all pregnancies end in miscarriage before twelve weeks, but miscarriage rates increase with a woman's age.

Mother's helper: Caretaker who cares for the child while the primary caretaker (mother or father) is close by or at home.

NICU (neonatal intensive care unit): Area of the hospital for ill or premature newborns.

OB-GYN (obstetrics and gynecology): An obstetrician delivers babies; a gynecologist specializes in women's health and treats diseases of reproductive organs. An OB-GYN does both.

Open adoption: Adoption where there is some degree of contact between birth parents and adoptive parents; can be "wide open" and include exchanging contact information and in-person visits or more limited, such as simply exchanging letters and photos as the child grows up.

PPD (post-partum depression): Condition affecting one out of eight new mothers, either before or after birth. A mood disorder, its symptoms include depression, including change in appetite, low energy, no interest in sex, and lack of sleep.

Pre-eclampsia: Usually occurring after 20 weeks of pregnancy and affecting 5 to 8 percent of all pregnancies, pre-eclampsia occurs only during pregnancy and impacts mothers and unborn babies. Marked by high blood pressure, swelling, headaches, and vision problems.

Placental problems: Any problem that impacts the placenta, which is attached to the uterus and is the lifeline between the mother and her unborn baby. Includes placenta abrupta (it pulls away from the uterus), placenta previa (placenta blocks the cervix) or placenta accreta (the placenta is attached too firmly to the uterus).

Prematurity: The term for babies born before 37 weeks of gestation, which can lead to negative outcomes such as heart defects, blindness, respiratory problems, or brain damage.

Primary infertility: When a couple that has no other biological children is unable to conceive or carry a pregnancy to term.

Progesterone-in-oil injections: Often used during ART. When a woman's natural progesterone level is insufficient, this is injected intramuscularly to prepare the uterus for a fertilized egg or embryo.

RAD (reactive attachment disorder): Condition that affects children who have learned that the world is unsafe and that adults are untrustworthy, leading to isolation from others. Children may be angry, emotional, or violent.

RE (reproductive endocrinologist): Type of doctor that specializes in fertility treatments. Board-certified as an OB/GYN doctor, an RE also has additional experience obtained from a fellowship in infertility.

Secondary infertility: The inability for a couple who already have a biological child (or children) to conceive or sustain a subsequent pregnancy. According to the National Center for Health Statistics, infertility impacts more than 3 million American women who already have had one or more successful pregnancies.

Selective reduction: Most commonly performed between 9 and 12 weeks of a pregnancy with multiples, the procedure involves injecting one or more fetuses with a chemical solution (potassium chloride) to stop the heartbeat.

Surrogate: A woman who volunteers to become pregnant on behalf of someone else, carrying her biological embryo or donor embryo. (Also see Gestational surrogate.)

TTC (tried to conceive): Acronym for how long someone's been struggling with infertility.

Unexplained infertility: A condition where no diagnosis can be reached as to the reason a man, woman, or couple is unable to conceive/maintain a healthy pregnancy. It impacts 20 percent of couples.

Uterine fibroids: Tumors or growths within the wall of the uterus. About 80 percent of women have them, and 25 percent of women experience severe pain and seek treatment. Can cause or be linked to infertility.

Index

bottle versus breastfeeding, 59–60

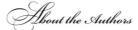
About the Authors

Jill S. Browning is a full-time mother of triplets, thanks to fertility treatments. She's also a freelance writer who specializes in subjects related to parenting. A contributing writer to *Chicago Parent* magazine, she has written articles for *Parenting* and the *Christian Science Monitor.*

Kelly James-Enger is the mother of a two-year-old son through domestic open adoption. She has written eight books, including *Small Changes, Big Results: A 12-Week Action Plan to a Better Life,* and more than seven hundred articles for national magazines, including *Family Circle, Health, Redbook,* and *Woman's Day.*

We'd love to hear from you! Please go to www.belatedbaby.com *and share your story of how infertility has impacted your parenting experience.*